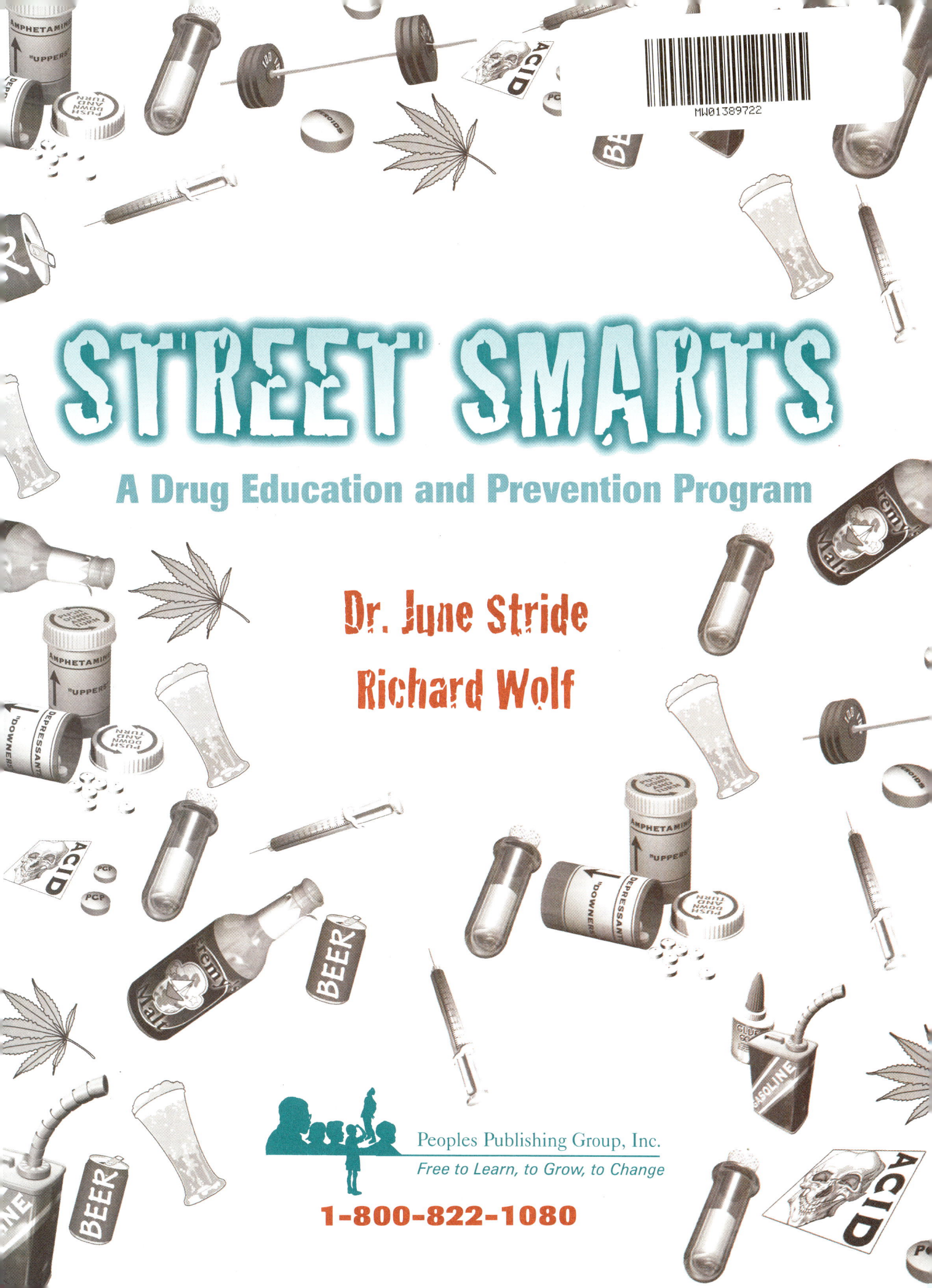

STREET SMARTS

A Drug Education and Prevention Program

Dr. June Stride

Richard Wolf

Peoples Publishing Group, Inc.
Free to Learn, to Grow, to Change

1-800-822-1080

Editor, *Charmaine Harris-Stewart*

Production Manager, *Doreen Smith*

Copy Editor, *Christine Cannistraro*

Proofreading, *Alida Mancinelli*

Cover Design, *Jeremy Mayes*

Design, *Jeremy Mayes, Michele Sakow*

Illustrations, *William Schmidt, Cara Ricioppo, Nick Massios, Armando Baéz, Jeremy Mayes*

Production/Electronic Design, *Janet Kliesch, Michele Sakow*

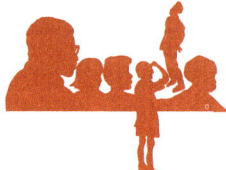

DEDICATION
Dedicated to Harriet Fleisher, educator, friend, mentor

ISBN 1-56256-723-3

© 1999

The Peoples Publishing Group, Inc.
230 W. Passaic Street
Maywood, New Jersey 07607

All rights reserved. No part of this book, excluding the SADD contracts on page iii and page iv and The Personal Growth Worksheet on page 119-120, may be kept in an information storage or retrieval system, transmitted or reproduced in any form or by any means without prior written permission of the Publisher.

Printed in the United States of America.

10 9 8 7 6 5 4 3 2

Street Smarts is fun.....Street Smarts is challenging...Street Smarts is uplifting...

ABOUT STREET SMARTS

Welcome to the Street Smarts substance abuse prevention program designed for adolescents and children of all ages. The program's unique, interactive format was developed, field-tested and revised over a ten-year period to respond to the realities and temptations that contribute to substance abuse. It utilizes drug education guidelines established by the federal government as well as recommendations from the latest national research.

Street Smarts interactive format goes far beyond cognitive information. Through use of a story line, positive role models, interpretive cartoons, cooperative learning and ethical decision-making activities, the program focuses on the underlying issue of drug-proofing behavior. It provides students with the knowledge and "Street Smarts" necessary to resist temptation. The program also challenges students to become proactive for themselves and for others.

DRUG-PROOFING BEHAVIOR

FEATURES

Many of the characteristic features of substance abuse are incorporated into thirteen vignettes organized by drug category. Each chapter begins with a provocative vignette that addresses issues of drug abuse within an ethical context. Each vignette utilizes a story within a story framework to provide positive role models to guide student thinking. Two main characters, Sergeant Leguero and Mrs. D., provide a safe environment for abusers to confront their drug problem and work toward proactive solutions for themselves and others.

Chapters are developmental and designed to support teachers and students in traditional or cooperative learning environments encouraging a variety of experiences: role play, individual or group projects and dramatic presentations that can be video recorded. Information about each drug is organized on **TELL IT** pages that provide factual information and **SHOW IT** pages that graphically depict the effects. The **HOOK, LINE, AND SINKER** page uses interpretive cartoons to show how people can get hooked, the lines (lies) that tempt people, and the sinkers then can lead to an abuser's downfall. On the **CHECKUP** page, matching, multiple choice and fill-the-blank questions provide a fun review and immediate feedback to students and teachers. A three-part interactive student page, **TAKE A STAND** allows students to recognize temptations and role-play ethical decision-making skills. The **YOUR TURN** page allows students to combine critical thinking skills with ethical decision making skills to make responsible choices.

Reproducibles   Reproducibles   Reproducibles

Supplemental materials for the Street Smarts program are offered in the *Street Smarts Teachers Edition*. They include crossword puzzles, ethical word searches, teaching suggestions and three reproducible unit reviews. The Street Smarts program concludes with a comprehensive end-of-book review and answer key.

Before you begin, take some time to review the SADD contracts on the following pages. SADD (Students Against Destructive Decisions) is a national organization committed to reducing unnecessary accidents and death by promoting substance-free lifestyles. SADD encourages open communication between teens and parents/guardians in which both pledge to share concerns about illegal substances and to sign a contract in which both promise to abstain.

Teens Agree:
1. To avoid alcohol and drugs.
2. To never drive under the influence of drugs or ride with a driver under the influence of drugs.
3. To call home for safe transportation to avoid an unsafe situation.
4. To buckle up for safety.

Parents/Guardians Agree:
1. To provide safe transportaion at any time of the day or night.
2. Not to ask questions, lecture, or discuss the situation until the situaiton can be discussed calmly.
3. Never to drive while under the influence or ride with any driver under the influence.
4. To buckle up for safety.

Join the SADD team!

Dr. June Stride

Richard Wolf

WORKING TOGETHER

In many states, parents/guardians, schools and teens are working together to help bring more public awareness to the problem of drinking and driving. Organizations like MADD (Mothers Against Destructive Decisions) and SADD (Students Against Destructive Decisions) have been fighting for tougher substance abuse enforcement laws. Many parent-teacher associations have invited guest speakers from these organizations into the schools. Parents and guardians often pledge to be home for all teen parties and to call other parents to assure alcohol/drug-free supervision. Many teens and their parents/guardians sign a contract (provided by SADD), that allows teens to call home for a ride at any time, no questions asked. Parents agree to hold off one day before discussing what happened. By working together, parents/guardians, schools and teens can become proactive in reducing unnecessary death and injury.

Read and discuss the contracts below with your parent/guardian. Join the team. Reduce unnecessary death.

Two contracts have been provided for your convenience. Middle School students may use the appropriate contract. Older students and non-student groups may use the generic contract.

CONTRACT FOR LIFE
STUDENTS AGAINST DESTRUCTIVE DECISIONS

A Contract for Life Between Parent and Middle School Student

Middle School Student:

I agree to learn as much as possible about the effects of illegal substances, to share with you my concerns about peer pressure, and to discuss these issues openly with you. I will contact you immediately for advice and guidance if I ever find myself in a situation where illegal substances are present. Under this contract I make a commitment to you not to use illegal substances. I also agree that I will not accept a ride with anyone who is under the influence of drugs or alcohol. I also agree to always "Buckle Up" and encourage others to do the same.

_____
Signature

Parent or Guardian:

I will seek information and educate myself about realities of illegal substances. I agree to be an ever-available resource for advice and communication with you. I agree that I will not use illegal substances. I also agree to seek safe, sober transportation home if I am ever in a situation where I have had too much to drink or a friend who is driving me has had too much to drink. I also agree to always wear my seat belt and encourage others to do the same.

_____   _____
Signature   Date

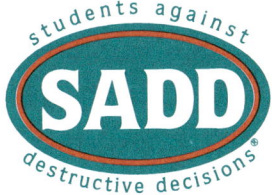

Students Against Destructive Decisions • Inc.

SADD and all SADD logos are registered with the United States Patent and Trademark Office and other jurisdictions. All rights reserved by SADD, Inc. a Massachusetts non-profit corporation. SADD, Inc. sponsors Students Against Driving Drunk, Students Against Destructive Decisions and other health and safety programs.

SADD, Inc., P.O. Box 800, Marlborough, MA 01752, Tel. 508-481-3568 • 508-945-3122

CONTRACT FOR LIFE
A Foundation for Trust and Caring

This contract is designed to facilitate communication between young people and their parents about potentially destructive decisions related to alcohol, drugs and violence. The issues facing young people today are often too difficult to address alone. SADD believes that effective parent-child communication is critically important in helping young adults to make healthy decisions.

Young Adult:

I recognize that there are many potentially destructive decisions I face every day and commit to you that I will do everything in my power to avoid making decisions that will jeopardize my health, safety, or your trust in me. I understand the dangers associated with the use of alcohol and drugs and the destructive behaviors often associated with impairment.

By signing below, I pledge my best effort to remain alcohol and drug-free and agree that I will never drive under the influence of either, or accept a ride from someone who is impaired.

Finally, I agree to call you if I am ever in a situation that threatens my safety and to communicate with you regularly about issues of importance to us both.

_____
Student

Parent (or Caring Adult):

I am committed to you, and to your health, and your safety. By signing below, I pledge to do everything in my power to understand and communicate with you about the many difficult and potentially destructive decisions you face.

Further, I agree to provide safe, sober transportation home if you are ever in a situation that threatens your safety and to defer discussion about that situation until a time when we can both discuss the issues in a calm and caring manner.

I also pledge to you that I will not drive under the influence of alcohol or drugs and will always seek safe, sober transportation home.

_____
Parent (or Caring Adult)

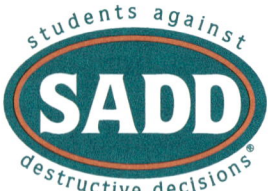

Students Against Destructive Decisions • Inc.

SADD and all SADD logos are registered with the United States Patent and Trademark Office and other jurisdictions. All rights reserved by SADD, Inc. a Massachusetts non-profit corporation. SADD, Inc. sponsors Students Against Driving Drunk, Students Against Destructive Decisions and other health and safety programs.

SADD, Inc., P.O. Box 800, Marlborough, MA 01752, Tel. 508-481-3568 • 508-945-3122

TABLE OF CONTENTS

Each chapter contains a realistic scenario or vignette, 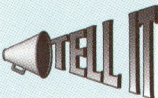 informational page(s), 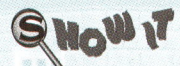 illustrations that graphically depict the effects of substance abuse, HOOK, LINE, AND SINKER interpretive cartoons, 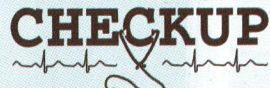 cognitive review, 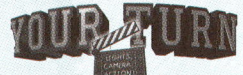 role play and ethical decision-making activities, 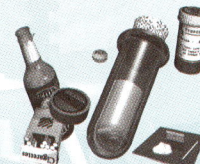 and critical thinking skills.

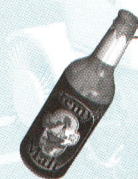
Chapter 1
DRUG ABUSE **1**

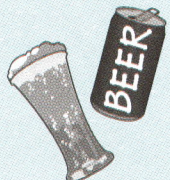
Chapter 2
ALCOHOL ABUSE **11**

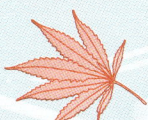
Chapter 5
MARIJUANA **39**

Chapter 3
ALCOHOL DEPENDENCE **20**

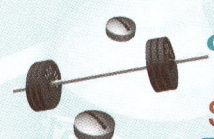
Chapter 6
STEROIDS **47**

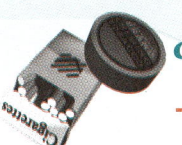
Chapter 4
TOBACCO **30**

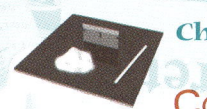
Chapter 7
COCAINE **55**

v

TABLE OF CONTENTS

Each chapter contains a realistic scenario or vignette, 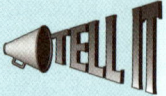 informational page(s), 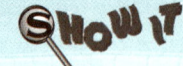 illustrations that graphically depict the effects of substance abuse, 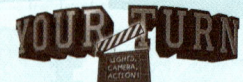 interpretive cartoons, 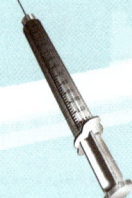 cognitive review, 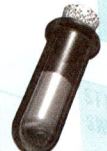 role play and ethical decision-making activities, 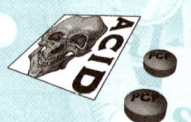 and critical thinking skills.

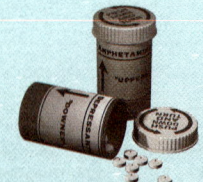

Chapter 8
CRACK 63

Chapter 9
HEROIN 72

Chapter 10
AMPHETAMINES
DEPRESSANTS 81

Chapter 11
INHALANTS 90

Chapter 12
OVER THE COUNTER/
PRESCRIPTION DRUGS 99

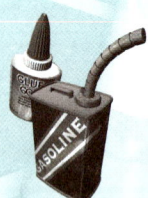

Chapter 13
HALLUCINOGENS 108

VI

DRUG ABUSE

CHAPTER 1

SECOND CHANCE

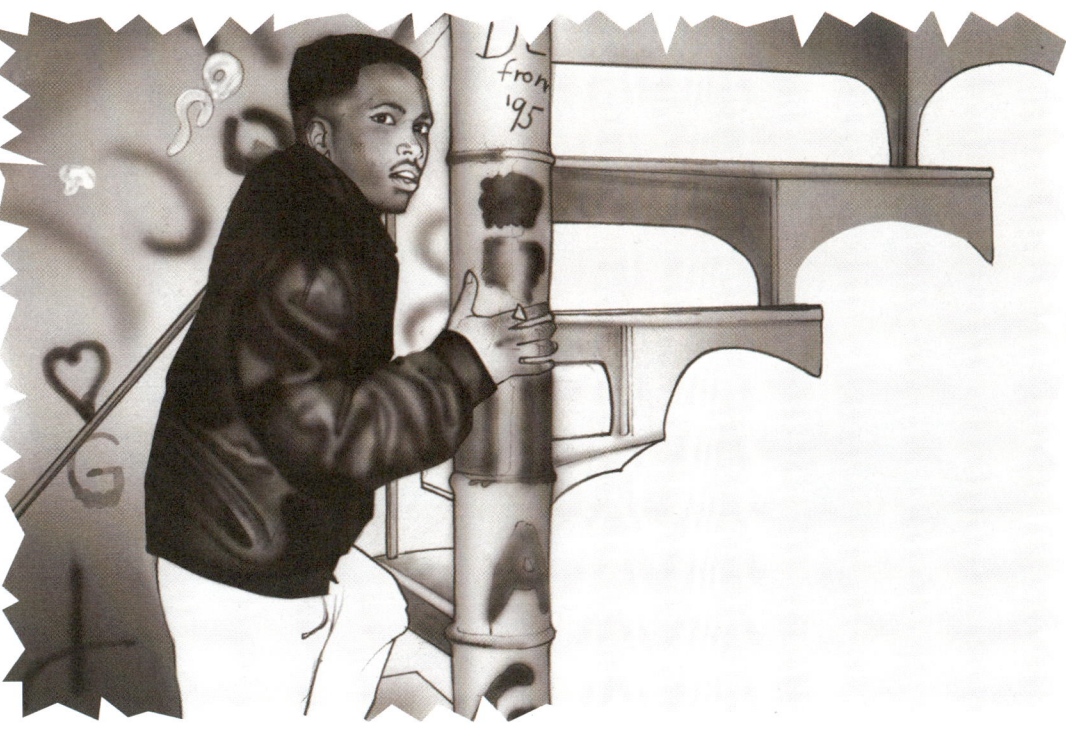

"This is it. It's now or never."

Derrick was running hard, in and out of yards, ducking behind fences and bushes. He knew they were after him. "Some friends!" he thought. "If they catch me, I'm dead!" He paused for a minute and listened. Maybe he had lost them.

As he turned the corner, he tripped and fell over an old garbage can. Several bags of marijuana flew out of his jacket pocket. His heart pounded as he sifted through the pile of garbage for the bags and stuffed them back into his pocket. Before he could catch his breath, shots rang out. They were closing in on him!

"How am I going to get out of this mess?" Derrick wondered, searching the block for a place to hide. A few feet ahead was a deserted stairwell. "This is it," he thought. "It's now or never."

Trapped

Derrick ducked into the stairwell and looked to see if anyone was following. The relief on his face turned to horror: two police officers were coming down the steps from the second floor landing. From their radios, he could hear the dispatcher's voice "... black male, between twelve and fifteen years old, wearing a black leather jacket..." Derrick turned to run, but he could hear the

THE PEOPLES PUBLISHING GROUP, 1-800-822-1080. COPYING PROHIBITED BY LAW.

1

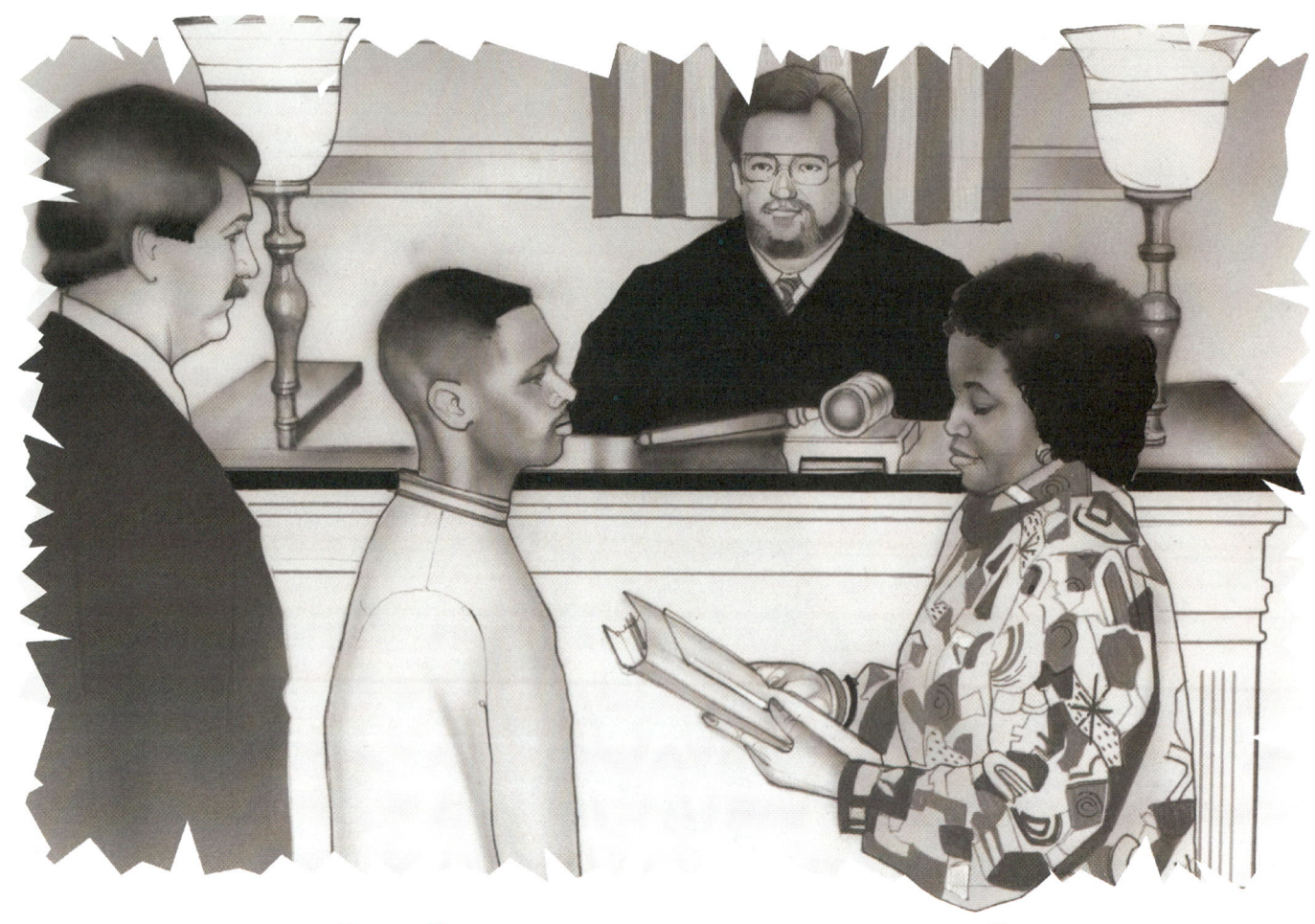

"YOU'RE GETTING A SECOND CHANCE."

wail of sirens on the street. He was trapped.

The Hearing

Derrick appeared in court neatly dressed. His clean-cut appearance showed no evidence of the "street smart" kid who had turned himself into the police. Judge Green, an ex-cop and former lawyer, peered down at Derrick from the bench. Derrick shivered under his cold stare. His life was in Judge Green's hands.

He doesn't look like the type to give a kid a break, Derrick thought. What if he's not as fair as everyone says he is?

"Well, I wondered when I'd see you in my court. Never figured it would be because you turned yourself in. How old are you now?" Judge Green asked in a deep voice.

Derrick, puzzled by the question, answered, "Fourteen, next birthday."

"I guess you and your friends were trying to make sure you wouldn't make it to fourteen. Is that what you want, son? Let me know. We can put you back on the street."

Derrick couldn't speak. He could only shake his head.

The judge motioned to a couple in the back of the courtroom. "Derrick, this is Sergeant Leguero and Mrs. D., they are going to make sure that you put your lifestyle of drugs and violence behind you. They work with a teen drug rehabilitation group called the "No-Mores.""

Mrs. D. walked over to Derrick and looked him

2 DRUG ABUSE Street Smarts

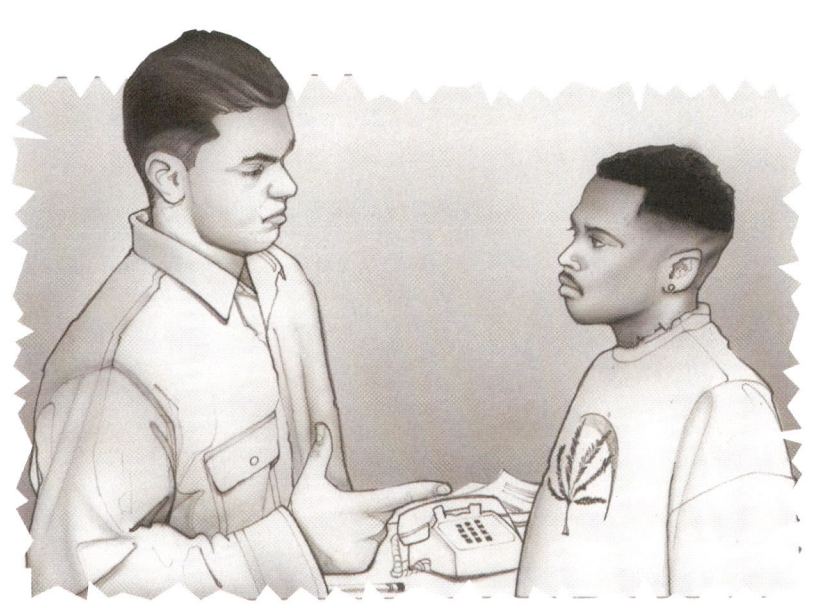

"...TAKE OFF THE SHIRT OR TURN IT INSIDE OUT."

straight in the face. "Derrick" she said, "You're getting a chance to join the "No-Mores" and turn things around for yourself. The sergeant and I set up the rules. You follow them exactly or faster than you can believe, you'll be back to Judge Green."

The sergeant added, "We meet Tuesdays and Fridays no questions, no excuses. You will be there. You will be part of the "No-Mores" and learn to like it. You don't understand something, you need advice or help, we're there for you. So is the group. You've got a new family."

A New Start

It was Derrick's first official meeting with the "No-Mores." He put on his favorite weed T-shirt. A smirk tugged at his lips as he stroked the large decal marijuana plant spread out across his chest. He looked at himself approvingly in the mirror. "I've got to hang with these "No-Mores" kids for awhile, but I don't have to turn into a geek." Derrick figured he'd play everyone until they got comfortable, then he would do his own thing.

Carlos, one of the long-term "No-Mores" members, watched Derrick stroll in; then he noticed his shirt.

Confrontation

Carlos exploded, "What's up with you, man? We're working hard to stay clean. Then you come in here mocking us, making like you're cool and drugs are cool."

All eyes were on Derrick.

"You know we ain't goin' let you in with no weed on your chest. You better take off the shirt or turn it inside out," a voice called out from the back of the room.

Mrs. D. and Leguero watched the confrontation between Derrick and the group in silence. Leguero, sensing that Derrick needed a chance to save face, called the meeting to order. As the group moved forward to take their seats, Derrick slipped quietly out of the room.

> "THE GREATEST QUEST IN LIFE IS TO REACH ONE'S POTENTIAL."
>
> *Michael Wynn*
> (Don't Quit)

TELL IT

Early Drug Use

The story of drug use and abuse can be traced back to early civilizations times. Early people had unusual qualities. found that certain plants Some had leaves that made their pain go away. Some had roots that, if boiled in water, made a tea or broth that caused people to relax or sleep. Other plants killed infection when placed on the affected area. People were chosen to keep the secrets of the plants. These "medicine people" used the secrets of plants to heal the sick.

Drug Use Today

Today much of the mystery about healing is gone. News reports tell us the latest medical discoveries. But people can still get wrong ideas about medicines. Some ads can make you believe that you can buy a pill to cure every ache and pain. Drugs are not the only cure. When people turn to drugs to "fix" all their problems, they end up with a bigger problem: drug abuse.

Uses and Abuses

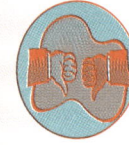

A drug is a substance that changes the way that the cells and tissues in your body work. Legal drugs called medicines are prescribed by doctors. Laws regulate their use to protect people from getting the wrong drug or the wrong amount of the drug.

Stores and pharmacies can sell some medicines, such as aspirin and cold remedies, without a prescription. These are called "over-the-counter" (OTC) drugs.

Street drugs are illegal drugs that are unregulated, not prescribed and against the law. Unlicensed and deadly, they are sold on the street, in homes, and anywhere people will buy. The ingredients and strength of these illegal drugs are not known. Often, to make more profit, street sellers mix in other ingredients (cut) with the street drug making the effects even more unpredictable. Use of street drugs is very dangerous.

Any drug can be abused. Misuse of an OTC drug or prescribed legal drug can result in injury or death. Improper use of such drugs include: overdose (taking too much or too often), taking a drug that is meant for another, taking a drug incorrectly (with the wrong food or liquid or at the wrong time), or using them after the expiration date. A person who uses drugs for no medical reason is considered a drug abuser.

Finding Help

Drug abuse hurts the abuser, the abuser's family, and many innocent people with whom the abuser comes into contact. Recovery from abuse cannot start until the abuser recognizes the problem and seeks help. Individual counseling and guided participation in groups with people with similar problems has helped many abusers overcome problems with drugs.

STREET SMART STRATEGIES

KNOWLEDGE POWER: Educate yourself about the proper use of medical drugs.
CORE VALUES: Recognize and avoid drug abuse situations.
PROACTION: Take a stand—practice drug abuse refusal skills.

BUZZ WORDS

1. Agitation — state of being upset
2. Cut — dilute or add "fillers" that stretch a drug
3. Drug — alters the way cells and tissues in the body work
4. Drug abuse — misuse of any drug
5. Dependent — unable to do without; to rely on something
6. Expiration date — latest date that medication can be used.
7. Hooked — dependent, addicted to a drug
8. Inappropriate — not proper
9. Medicine — a drug prescribed by a doctor or an over-the-counter drug taken for health reasons
10. Overdose — taking too much or too often
11. Over-the-counter (OTC) — legal drugs sold without prescription in a pharmacy
12. Prescribed — medicine ordered by a doctor with a doctor's note
13. Street drug — illegal drug; non-medical drug sold on street
14. Suspicious — feeling mistrust

SHOW IT

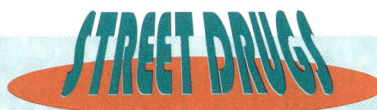 STREET DRUGS

People who make and sell street drugs are not interested in helping others; they are usually interested in making money for themselves. The ingredients and strength of these illegal drugs are not known. Often, to make more profit, street sellers mix in other ingredients (**cut**) with the street drug making the effects even more unpredictable. Use of street drugs is very dangerous.

WHO ARE THE ABUSERS?

INFANT/CHILD

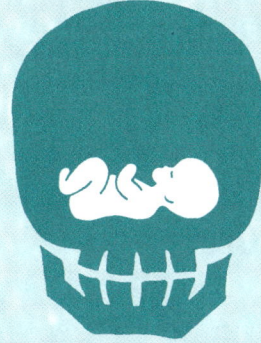

POSSIBLE REASON: Addiction passed on during pregnancy or infancy

POTENTIAL RISK: Brain damage, retardation, physical problems, death

TEEN

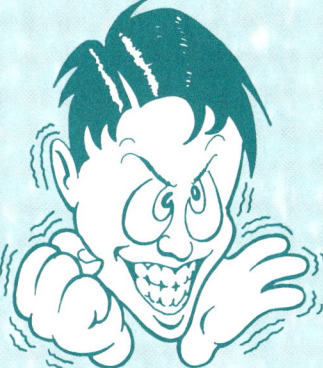

POSSIBLE REASON: Peer pressure, desire to belong, curiosity, adventure, rebellion, escape from reality, improved athletic performance

POTENTIAL RISK: Physical and psychological dependence, physical and mental damage, death, high risk for violence, STDs, AIDS, pregnancy, crime, legal or family problems, inability to concentrate causing school or job problems

ADULT

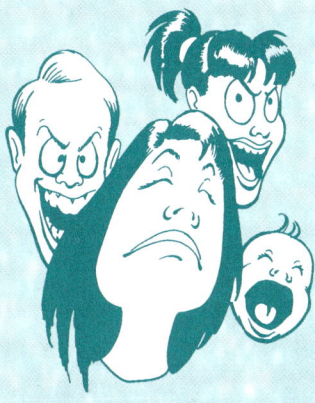

POSSIBLE REASON: Peer pressure, stress of job or family, curiosity, escape from reality, quick "fix" to problems

POTENTIAL RISK: Family/job related problems, passing addiction to an unborn child, potential for child/spouse abuse, violent behavior, crime and legal problems

ELDERLY

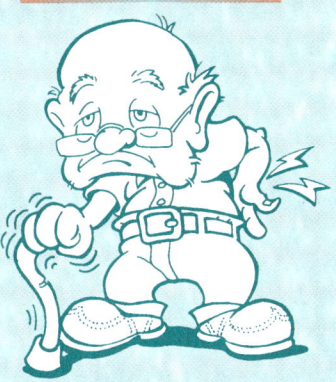

POSSIBLE REASON: Loneliness, pain, improperly prescribed medicine, accident due to poor vision, memory, diet

POTENTIAL RISK: Physical and psychological dependence, physical and mental damage, death, becoming more fragile and therefore more at risk of abuse by others, inability to care for self

Anyone can become a drug abuser! Regardless of their background, sex, color, ethnicity, or age, people can develop problems with drugs. Indeed, some people are abusers but either don't know it or constantly deny that they have a problem. When people become **hooked** or addicted to a drug, they have become **dependent** upon the drug. Regular use of the drug is no longer an option for them: it has become a necessity.

SHOW IT: RECOGNIZING DRUG ABUSE

How can you recognize if you or someone you know has a drug problem? If you are unsure if you have a problem, more than likely you do. If a friend or family member begins to show one or more of the following signs of changed behavior, it may mean a drug abuse problem. Or, it may indicate that there is some other problem that needs attention.

Signs of Possible Drug Abuse

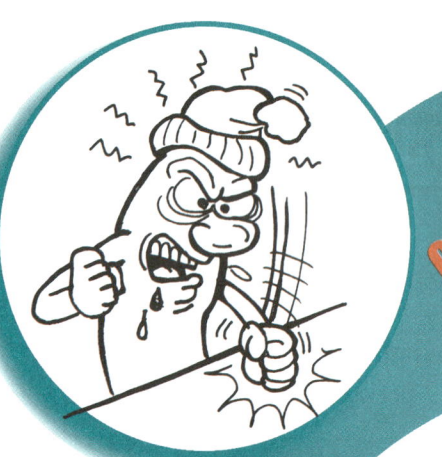
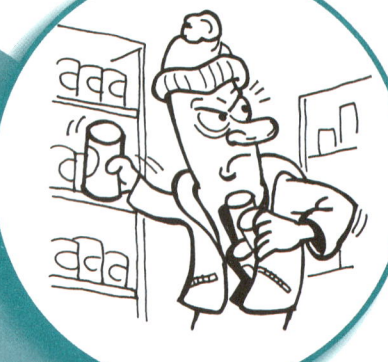
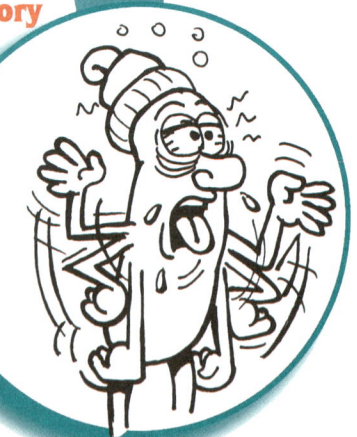

- stealing
- sudden behavior change
- sudden physical change
- rapid mood swings
- violent/inappropriate behavior
- slurred speech, poor coordination, loss of memory
- depression/withdrawal/extreme agitation
- change in appearance
- lying, cheating
- change in circle of friends
- suspicious behavior

Co$t of Abu$e

Drug abusers need help. Their abuse affects not only themselves and their performance in school, work and the community, but family and friends as well. Increasing drug problems have resulted in increasing community crime, increasing school problems and increasing medical expenses. Just as serious to any country, state, community and family is the fact that drug dependence results in decreased ability to make a positive contribution to society. Each of us pays the price of drug abuse. Each of us has a responsibility to help stop drug abuse.

DRUG ABUSE — Street Smarts

HOOK, LINE, AND SINKER

HOOK: The drugs that get people hooked. **LINE:** The lie that gets them to take the drugs. **SINKER:** The bad results of taking drugs.

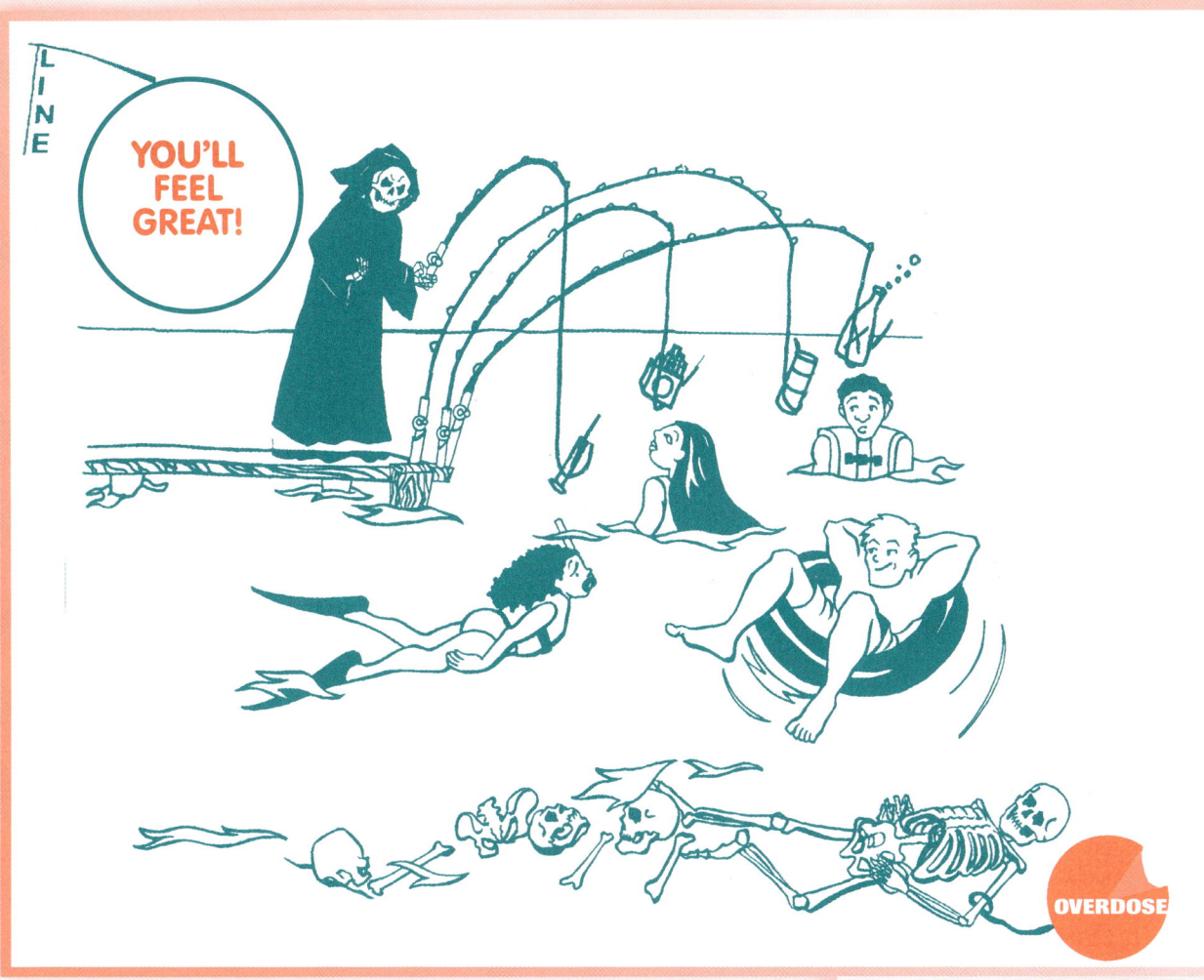

THINK ABOUT IT...

Use the cartoon above to answer the following questions:

HOOK — Name one drug an abuser might inject.
_____
_____

LINE — What line is tempting these swimmers?
_____
_____

SINKER — What killed the abuser?
_____
_____

Be Street Smart
Walk Away

For Advice And Information Call:
National Council on Alcoholism and Drug Dependence (NCADD)
1-800-NCA-Call
or
http://www.ncadd.org

THE PEOPLES PUBLISHING GROUP, 1-800-822-1080. COPYING PROHIBITED BY LAW.

7

CHECKUP

MATCHING

Column A   **Column B**

1. Over-the-counter drug
2. prescribed
3. drug abuser
4. expired
5. inappropriate

a. anyone who misuses any type of drug
b. finished, no longer good
c. OTC drug
d. not correct
e. especially designed for someone

FILL IN THE BLANKS

crime   drop out   all   job
anyone   deny   expensive   help

_____ can become a drug abuser. Some people are drug abusers and _____ that they have a problem. All drug abusers need _____. Drug abuse is _____. We _____ pay the price. Abusers may turn to _____ to pay for their habit. An abuser may _____ of school or lose their _____ because of behavior changes. Drug abusers sometimes abuse their family and friends.

MULTIPLE CHOICE

1. **Over-the-counter drugs**
   a. need a prescription
   b. are illegal
   c. can be purchased in a pharmacy without prescription

2. **Street drugs are**
   a. legal drugs
   b. over-the-counter drugs
   c. illegal drugs

3. **Prescription drugs**
   a. are illegal
   b. are over-the-counter drugs
   c. are given by a medical doctor.

4. **Drug abuse is**
   a. non-medical use of drug
   b. misuse of medical drug
   c. both a and b

5. **Recognizing the signs of drug abuse can**
   a. help you help yourself
   b. help you help others
   c. both a and b

DRUG ABUSE — Street Smarts

TAKE A STAND

Dear Mrs. D.

IMPROVE YOUR REFUSAL SKILLS

Dear Mrs. D.:
  I'm a pudge. My friends tell me I'm fat. My parents tell me I'm just right. I know they say that so as not to hurt my feelings.
  All my friends are trim and can wear the latest styles. I look like a tank in them. I hate looking at myself.
  Yesterday I decided I needed help to stop eating so much. I took my allowance and bought some diet pills. Now I'm afraid to use them. I'm writing to you because I've heard bad stories about people who have used diet pills. What do you recommend?

  Signed,
  Fat and tired of it.

Write how you would answer if you were Mrs. D.

Mrs. D. Answers:
_____
_____
_____
_____
_____
_____
_____
_____
_____

Show that you recognize the danger by completing the exercise below.

Timmy lives with his grandmother. He likes her a lot.
  They can really talk about most things but when it comes to "her medicine," there is no discussion.
  Every night Grandma takes the sleeping pills prescribed for Grandpa who died last year. Grandma is only 90 pounds and Grandpa weighed over 200 pounds. Grandma is not herself when she finally gets up in the morning, she doesn't seem to be able to concentrate. Timmy is afraid to leave her alone, even to go to school.

1. *Underline* a sentence that tells what Grandma is doing wrong.

2. (Circle) a line that shows how Grandma's behavior puts Timmy at risk.

3. LIST one positive step Timmy could take to improve the situation.
_____
_____

Write the coolest way to say, "No!"

1. **The Offer** "What do you say, James? I'm going to pop a few beers. Want to join me?"

   You say _____
   _____

2. **The Dare** "Dad will be home in a half-hour. I dare you to finish that bottle of wine before he gets in!"

   You say _____
   _____

   BACK OFF

3. **The Threat** "When you joined the sorority, you agreed to be part of what we do. If you don't go drinking with us tonight, you're out."

   You say _____
   _____

4. **The Feel Good Approach** "I have some anti-depressant pills left over from my therapist. You've been so low, why don't you try them?"

   You say _____
   _____

THE PEOPLES PUBLISHING GROUP, 1-800-822-1080. COPYING PROHIBITED BY LAW.

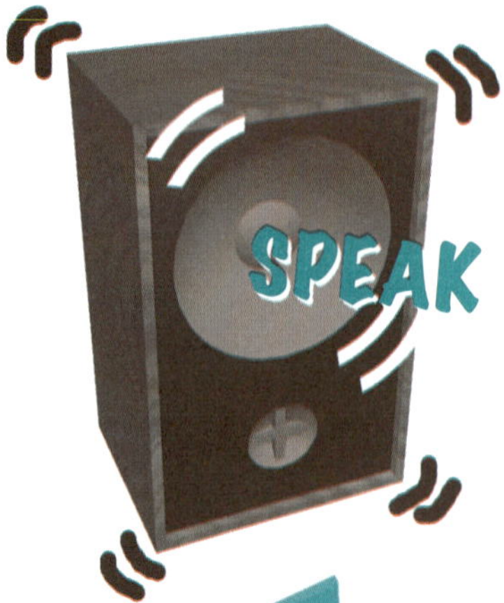

YOUR TURN

SPEAK OUT

LIGHTS, CAMERA, ACTION!

1. You know that many prescribed medicines have side effects but you are not sure about the side effects of the medicine prescribed for your family members. How would you go about checking out each medicine?

   _____
   _____

2. Old bottles, tubes and containers of medicines in closets and medicine cabinets are safety hazards. What is the best way to eliminate the threat?

   _____
   _____

PARENT — ASK AN ADULT GUARDIAN

ASK:
"Do you feel that people today are more likely to look for a short cut for curing illnesses than when you were growing up?"

"How has TV and advertising changed the way people think about drugs?"

INTERACT

Setting: You are on the school newspaper and have a reputation for reporting the truth.

Situation: Your school is obsessed with "thin." To be fat and popular is unheard of. To be chubby and popular is rare. You have heard about a serious problem with many girls taking diet pills or laxatives, especially those trying out for the cheerleader squad. You try not to embarrass anyone when you write your articles. You are afraid that certain girls will be made fun of if you tell this story, but you feel the story must be told for health reasons.

Solution: How will you handle the situation? If you write the article, what point of view will you take?

Teen Talk

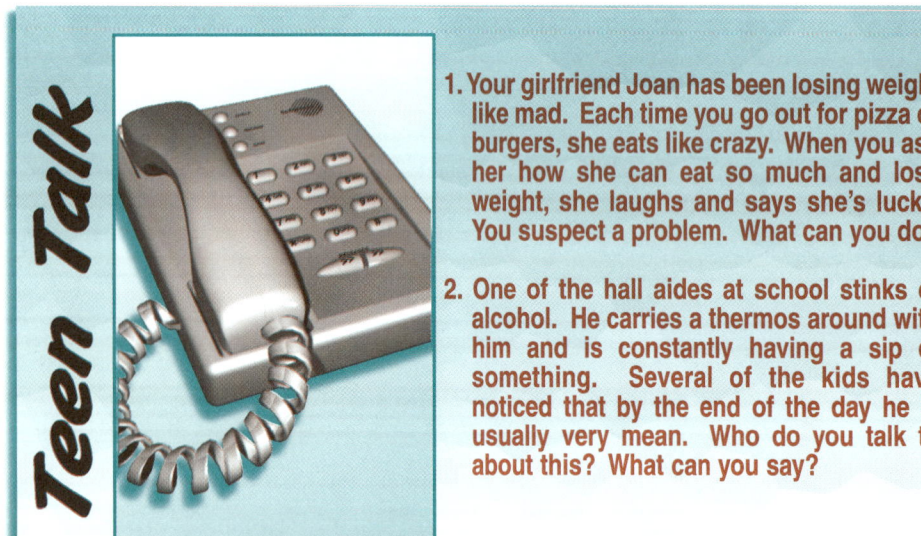

1. Your girlfriend Joan has been losing weight like mad. Each time you go out for pizza or burgers, she eats like crazy. When you ask her how she can eat so much and lose weight, she laughs and says she's lucky. You suspect a problem. What can you do?

2. One of the hall aides at school stinks of alcohol. He carries a thermos around with him and is constantly having a sip of something. Several of the kids have noticed that by the end of the day he is usually very mean. Who do you talk to about this? What can you say?

10   DRUG ABUSE   Street Smarts

ALCOHOL ABUSE
CHAPTER 2
TOTALLED

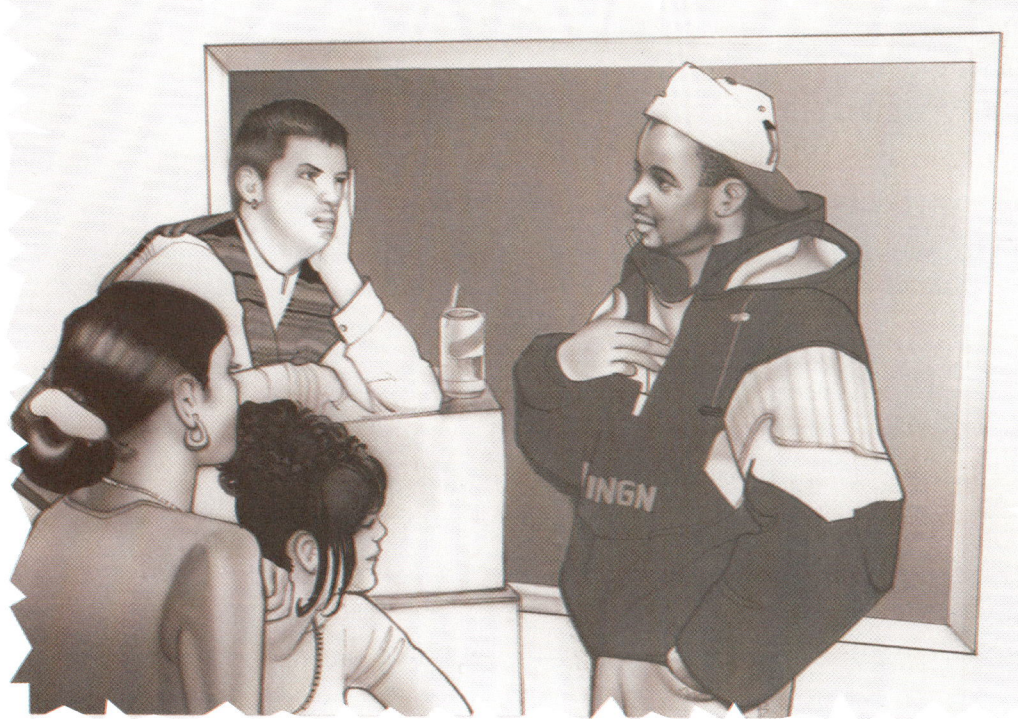

"I WAS JUST HAVING A LITTLE FUN. I DIDN'T MEAN FOR IT TO HAPPEN THAT WAY."

Bo took a deep breath and leaned against the wall. For weeks he had felt like an outsider at the "No-Mores" weekly meetings. Now he finally felt as if he belonged. He walked over to the table. It was his turn to tell his story.

Mrs. D. looked up and smiled. Bo cleared his throat and began.

"I started in sixth grade. I'd sneak a beer or some wine when my Moms wasn't home. Moms really never knew how much was there since her brother drank, too."

Juana called out. "I remember you in science class in junior high. When you weren't sleeping in class, you were making trouble. No matter what Mr. Hill said, you'd do something crazy to disrupt the lesson. We never knew what would happen when you were in class."

"I didn't hear you complaining. You were having as much fun as we were," said Bo evenly. "Anyway, I wasn't the only one who was wasted. All my buddies were drinking, too."

LaMonte interrupted, "Hey, Bo, didn't your mom suspect anything?"

Grounded

"My Moms complained that I spent too much time hanging out with my friends. But there was no way she could keep up with everything I was doing.

11

Between the divorce from my dad and working overtime nursing to pay the bills, she didn't get home before seven most nights. I had plenty of time to go through the mail and get rid of failure notices or discipline slips for cutting class. I got over for quite a while, but she finally insisted that I give her my report card. That did it! When she saw all the failing grades, she went crazy. I was grounded."

Mrs. D. spoke up, "Bo, there's something you're not telling us. You wouldn't be here if you hadn't gotten in trouble with the law."

"Yeah, well, it's not my favorite story. It happened in the beginning of 10th grade. The neighbors were away and Moms was watching their house and car for them. As usual, I was "grounded." The guys called. I could hear the music blasting in the background. They wanted to know why I was still home and not at the party. I glanced at the clock. It was only 8 P.M., Moms had the late shift at the hospital and wouldn't be home before midnight. I figured I could go to the party for a few hours, leave early and be back before she got home."

"Buzzed"

"I ran into the kitchen, grabbed the neighbor's car keys off the counter and took off. The party was slammin' when I got there, and I was way behind. Everyone was already buzzed. I figured vodka was the fastest way to catch up. Before I knew it, it was midnight."

"I jumped into the car and floored it. From the rear view mirror I could see this cop coming up fast behind me. There was only one exit to go. I thought I could make it. I turned the wheel for the exit, but somehow the car and I weren't communicating. The next thing I knew, people were trying to get me out of the car. The whole front end was hugging a tree. I guess the tree stopped the car."

Mrs. D. looked straight at Bo. "Let me get this straight, Bo. You disobeyed your mother and went out even though you were grounded, you took your neighbor's car without permission, you drove under the influence of alcohol, you ran from the police, *and* you totalled your neighbor's car. I *know* you don't expect my sympathy."

Bo was annoyed. "This stinks!" said Bo, voicing the irritation he felt at Mrs. D.'s words. "I thought you'd understand. Don't you get it? I was just having a little fun. I didn't mean for it to happen that way."

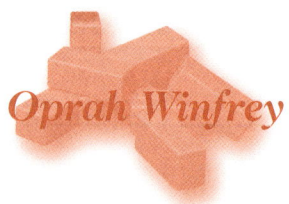

"NOT ONLY ARE YOU RESPONSIBLE FOR YOUR LIFE, BUT DOING THE BEST AT THIS MOMENT PUTS YOU IN THE BEST PLACE FOR THE NEXT MOMENT."

Oprah Winfrey

TELL IT

The Number One Drug Problem

Alcohol is the number-one drug problem in the United States. Alcoholic beverages are made from **fermented** or **distilled** fruits and grains. Sometimes alcoholic beverages, such as wine coolers, mislead drinkers by masking the **alcohol** taste with a fruit-like flavor. Drinkers mistakenly think that they can drink as much as they want without getting drunk. The term "light beer" is also misleading. Light beer has a reduced number of calories but not a reduced alcoholic content.

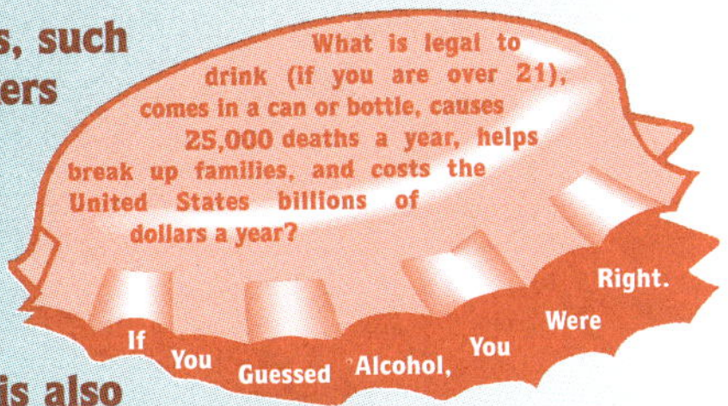

Drinking once in a while is called social drinking. If alcohol is taken in excess, however, drinking becomes a problem. Because alcohol is easy to get, and its use is accepted in many cultures, people sometimes go beyond social drinking without anyone even noticing.

What is legal to drink (if you are over 21), comes in a can or bottle, causes 25,000 deaths a year, helps break up families, and costs the United States billions of dollars a year? If You Guessed Alcohol, You Were Right.

The Waste of Getting Wasted

No matter how it is used, alcohol is **toxic** (poison); it affects everyone who drinks it.

As a **depressant**, it slows down the body's responses and functions. If too much alcohol is consumed at one time, it shuts down the part of the brain that controls breathing. The abuser dies from lack of oxygen caused by **alcohol poisoning**. Because alcohol affects judgment, people take greater risks when they're drinking. Accidents occur because alcohol slows reactions and blurs vision.

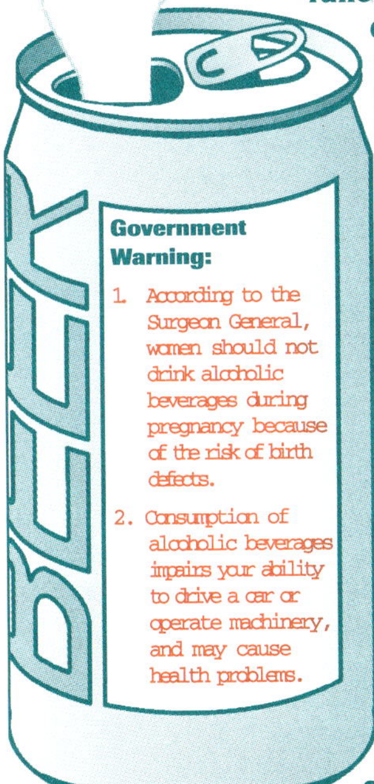

Government Warning:
1. According to the Surgeon General, women should not drink alcoholic beverages during pregnancy because of the risk of birth defects.
2. Consumption of alcoholic beverages impairs your ability to drive a car or operate machinery, and may cause health problems.

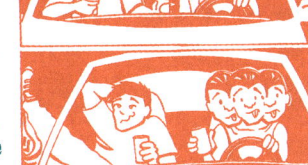

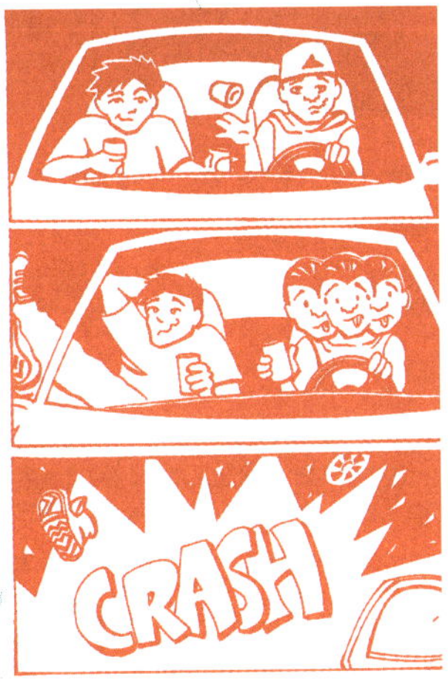

Stay Healthy—ABSTAIN

Experts caution "If you drink, don't drive. If you drive, don't drink." Never get into a vehicle whose driver has been drinking. You help yourself and you help others when you do not drink.

Many teens have joined an organization called **SADD**, Students Against Destructive Decisions. SADD does not approve of any drinking by anyone under the legal age. They sponsor school groups to encourage abstinence from alcohol. The organization has developed a contract, SADD Contract for Life, that teens and their parents sign. Teens agree that they will NEVER drive themselves or with anyone who has been drinking. Parents agree to arrange a ride home, NO questions asked (see pages iii and iv).

STREET SMART STRATEGIES

KNOWLEDGE POWER:
Learn how alcohol affects the mind and body.

CORE VALUES:
Have alcohol-free friends and alcohol-free fun.

PROACTION:
Take a stand—practice alcohol refusal skills. Don't drink.

BUZZ WORDS

1. **Abstain** — not do something
2. **Alcohol** — a drink that contains ethyl alcohol, an addicting drug
3. **Alcohol poisoning** — shuts off oxygen to the brain
4. **BAL or blood alcohol level** — measure of the amount of alcohol in a person's blood
5. **Chug** — drink heavily
6. **Depressant** — slows down brain and central nervous system
7. **Distilled** — process of heating that makes stronger alcohol, such as whiskey or vodka
8. **Drunk** — wasted; bombed; under the influence of alcohol
9. **Fermented** — process of using yeast with grains and fruits to make alcoholic beverages, such as beer or wine
10. **Hangover** — sick feeling that is the result of drinking too much
11. **Intoxicating** — causes a person to get drunk
12. **Liquor** — stronger alcohol than wine or beer because much of the water is taken out of the alcohol
13. **SADD** — organization of Students Against Destructive Decisions
14. **Sober** — not drunk
15. **Toxic** — poisonous

THE PEOPLES PUBLISHING GROUP, 1-800-822-1080. COPYING PROHIBITED BY LAW.

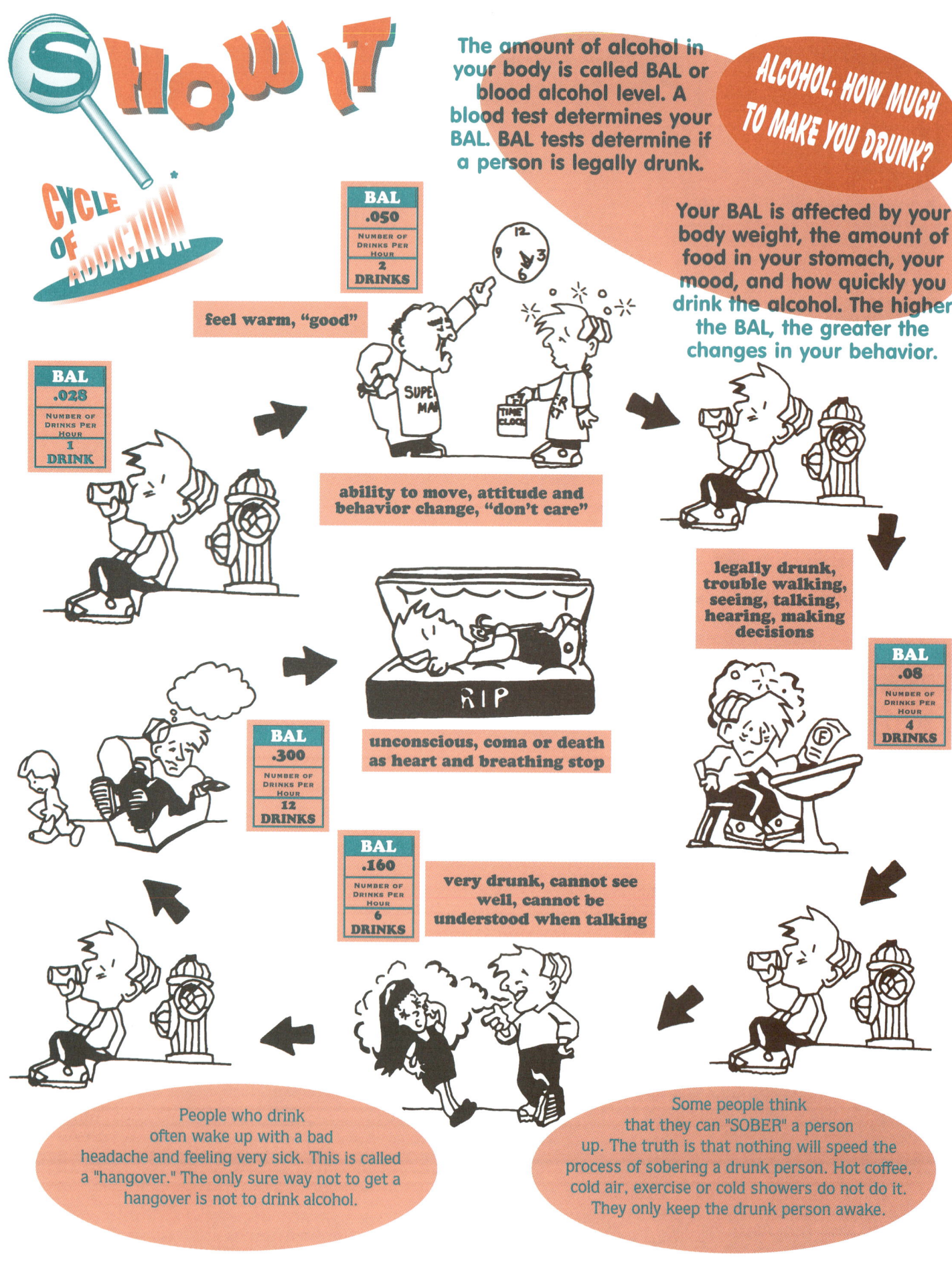

SHOW IT

WHAT WHERE WHEN WHY

Alcohol's effect on you is determined by its rate of absorption into the bloodstream. How quickly a person gets drunk depends upon the following:

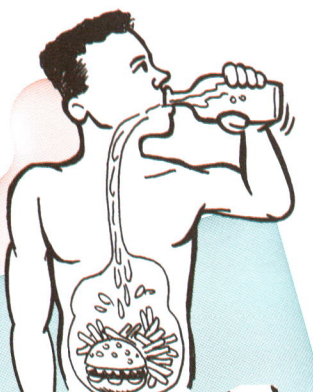

Food in Stomach
Eating before or while drinking delays the passage of alcohol into the blood. It does not stop it!

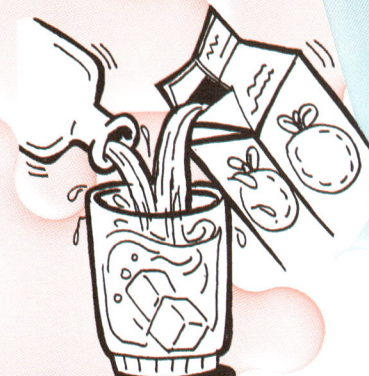

The Mix
When alcohol is mixed with other liquids, the rate of absorption changes. Water decreases the rate of absorption. Carbonated beverages increase the rate of absorption.

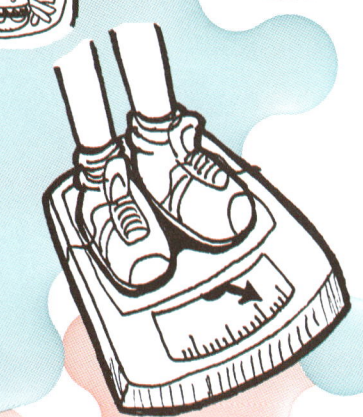

Weight
The less you weigh, the quicker the alcohol will be felt.

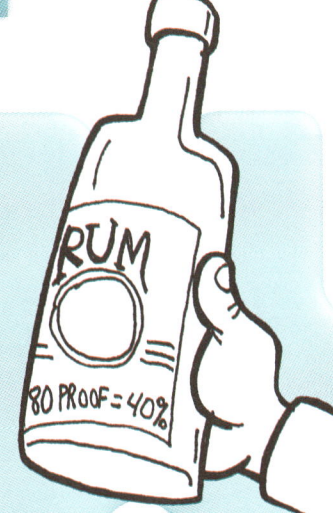

The Proof
The strength of ethyl alcohol is written on the side of the can or bottle (for example 80 proof is the same as 40% alcohol).

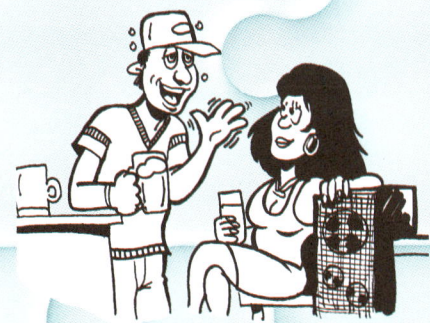

Set And Setting
The attitude of the drinker, the company the drinker is with, and the physical position of the drinker change the effect of alcohol. (An upset person, or one standing, may feel the effects of alcohol more quickly.)

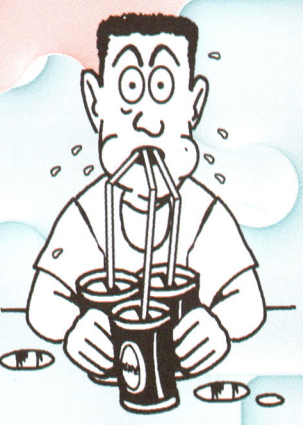

"Chug"
The quicker alcohol gets into the body the more time it takes for the liver to get rid of it.

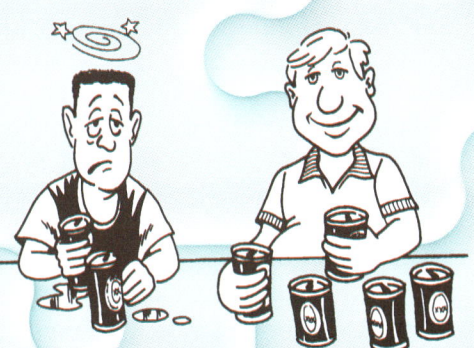

Tolerance
A person who has been exposed to alcohol before will not feel the effects of alcohol as quickly as a first time drinker. Some drinkers must drink more and more each time they drink to get the same effect.

THE PEOPLES PUBLISHING GROUP, 1-800-822-1080. COPYING PROHIBITED BY LAW.

HOOK, LINE, AND SINKER

HOOK: The drugs that get people hooked. **LINE:** The lie that gets them to take the drugs. **SINKER:** The bad results of taking drugs.

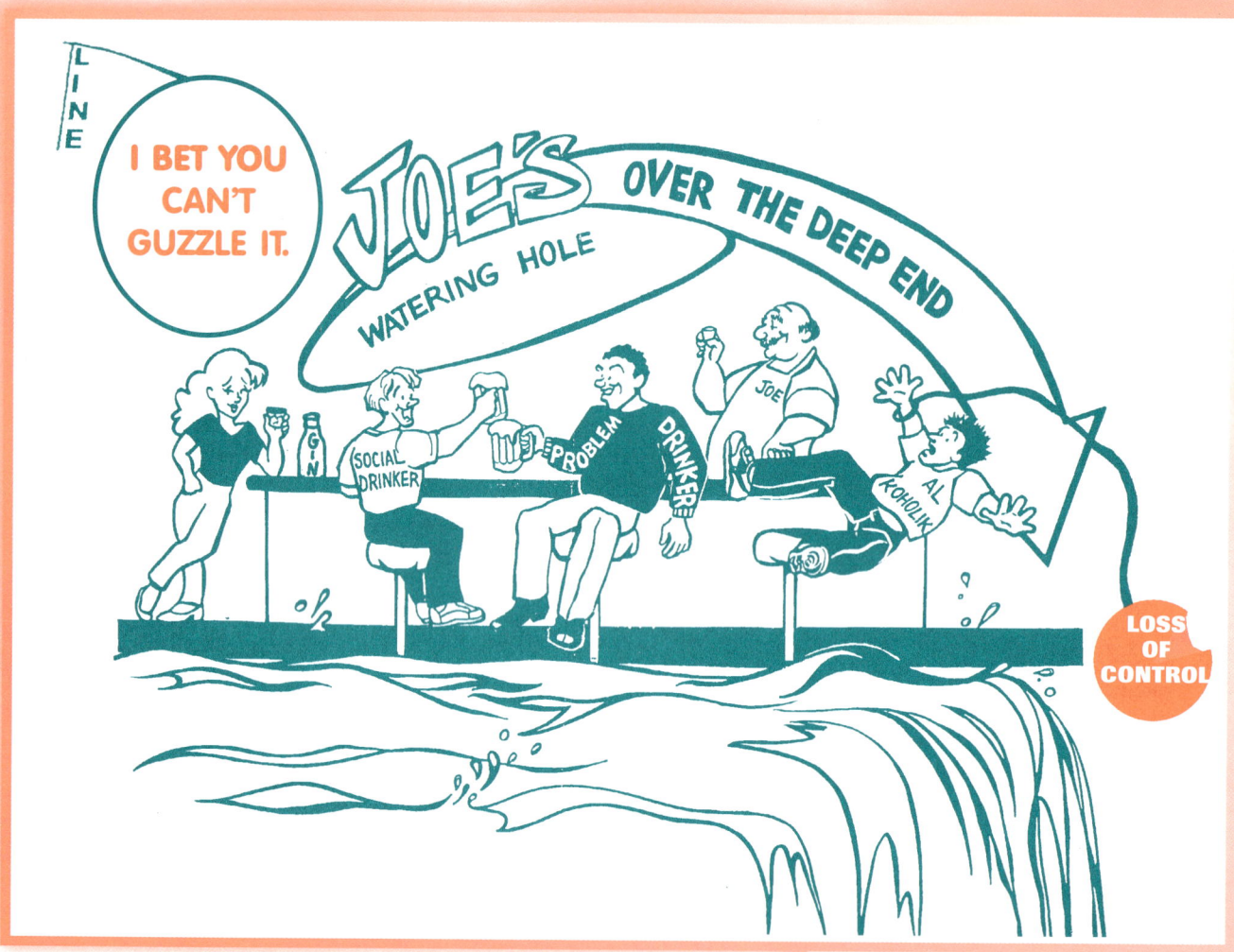

THINK ABOUT IT...

Use the cartoon above to answer the following questions:

What drug is being abused at Joe's?

_____
_____

What line is challenging these drinkers?

_____
_____

What is pulling Al Koholik over the deep end?

_____
_____

Be Street Smart

Walk Away

For Advice And Information Call:

National Council on Alcoholism and Drug Dependence (NCADD)

1-800-NCA-Call

or

http://www.ncadd.org

16   ALCOHOL ABUSE   Street Smarts

CHECKUP

MATCHING

Column A   Column B

1. ___ BAL   a. speed drinking
2. ___ alcohol   b. blood alcohol level
3. ___ sober   c. a liquid drug
4. ___ hangover   d. sick feeling caused from drinking too much
5. ___ chug   e. not drunk

FILL IN THE BLANKS

poor   alcohol   think
one   quickly   behavior

Beer, wine and liquor are all kinds of _____. Alcohol works _____ in the body because it is absorbed directly into the bloodstream. Alcohol changes _____ because it alters the way people _____. People who use alcohol may make _____ decisions. Alcohol is the number _____ drug problem in the United States.

MULTIPLE CHOICE

1. Which of the following sobers a person?
   a. coffee
   b. cold shower
   c. passage of time

2. Which person would most likely feel the effects of alcohol first?
   a. 100-pound teenager
   b. 150-pound teenager
   c. 125-pound adult

3. Which of these bad things could happen to a drunk driver?
   a. police arrest
   b. kill self or others
   c. both a & b

4. What is BAL?
   a. amount of alcohol in the blood
   b. balance
   c. a quick way to get drunk

5. An early sign of getting drunk is
   a. slowed speech
   b. unconsciousness
   c. coma

THE PEOPLES PUBLISHING GROUP, 1-800-822-1080. COPYING PROHIBITED BY LAW.

TAKE A STAND

Dear Mrs. D.

IMPROVE YOUR REFUSAL SKILLS

Dear Mrs. D.:
   Keith and I have been best buddies since third grade. We're in the tenth grade now. Every weekend he drinks. Either it's at a party or he gets a six-pack. After he has a few beers, he acts rude and loud. He thinks he's funny.
   I'm worried about him. I don't want to be around him when he drinks and I don't want to drink to stay friends with him. What should I do?

Signed,
Concerned But Annoyed

Write how you would answer if you were Mrs. D.

Mrs. D. Answers:
_____
_____
_____
_____
_____
_____
_____
_____
_____
_____

Show that you recognize the danger by completing the exercise below.

Mike's dad meets his high school buddies every weekend for a few beers. They plan big parties for their families at every holiday and hang around together drinking and telling "drunk" stories.
   Teenagers are allowed to have a few drinks at these get-togethers. Mike's father says he is looking forward to the time when Mike will "drink with the boys."

1. <u>Underline</u> two sentences that describe how Mike's father is putting Mike at risk.

2. (Circle) a line that shows how Mike's father and his buddies are encouraging teenagers to drink.

3. **LiSt** one thing that Mike and the other teens could do to change the tradition of drinking in their families.
_____
_____
_____
_____

Write the "coolest" way to say, "No!"

1. **The Offer** Your friend finds two beers left from his parents' party. He says, "Let's each have one."
   You say _____
   _____

2. **The Dare** It's your first date with Ricky. He says, "Don't tell me I'm out with a baby. Have a drink."
   You say _____
   _____

   BACK OFF

3. **The Threat** "If you back out of this beer drinking contest now, you'll never be able to show your face around here again."
   You say _____
   _____

4. **The Feel Good Approach** "A couple glasses of wine ad a hot bubble bath will make you feel a lot better about your break up with José."
   You say _____
   _____

ALCOHOL ABUSE — Street Smarts

SPEAK OUT

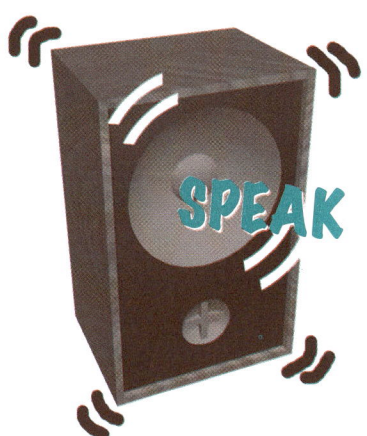

1. If you were a judge, how would you handle second time offenders arrested for driving while intoxicated? What type of community service might change the abuser's behavior?

_____
_____

2. You are a single parent of twin teenage boys who are both on the football team. What is the best way to help them abstain from alcohol?

_____
_____

PARENT ASK AN ADULT GUARDIAN

ASK:
Were any of your friends or families involved in accidents due to alcohol use? What happened?

INTERACT

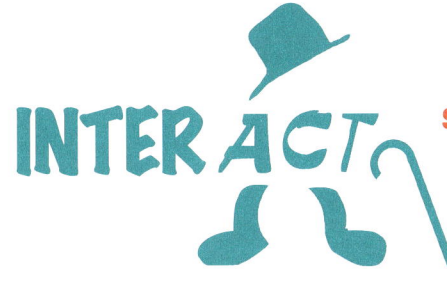

Setting: Your sister was killed two years ago on prom night. Her date insisted on driving even though he'd had too much to drink. He ran the car into a tree. You are now a member of Students Against Destructive Decisions (SADD). You want to stay alcohol-free.

Situation: All the kids in your crowd are putting pressure on you to "lighten up": they mean drink.

Solution: Act out the scene between you and your friends. Give several ways you can tell your friends "No."

Teen Talk

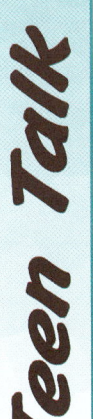
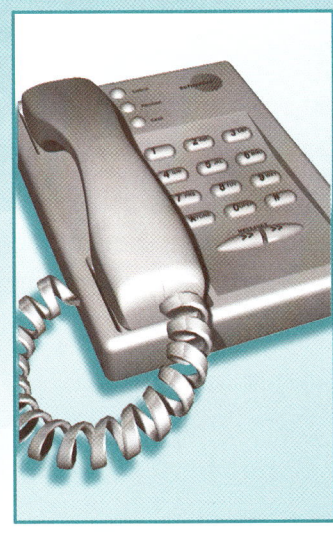

1. Amy's parents are going away for the weekend. Amy decides to have a slumber party so she won't be home alone. The word gets out at school that there will be a "bring your own booze" party at Amy's house. What can Amy do to stop a possible disaster?

2. What steps can you take to help your friend?

_____
_____
_____
_____
_____
_____
_____

THE PEOPLES PUBLISHING GROUP, 1-800-822-1080. COPYING PROHIBITED BY LAW.

CHAPTER 3: ALCOHOL DEPENDENCE

MIKE'S CHOICE

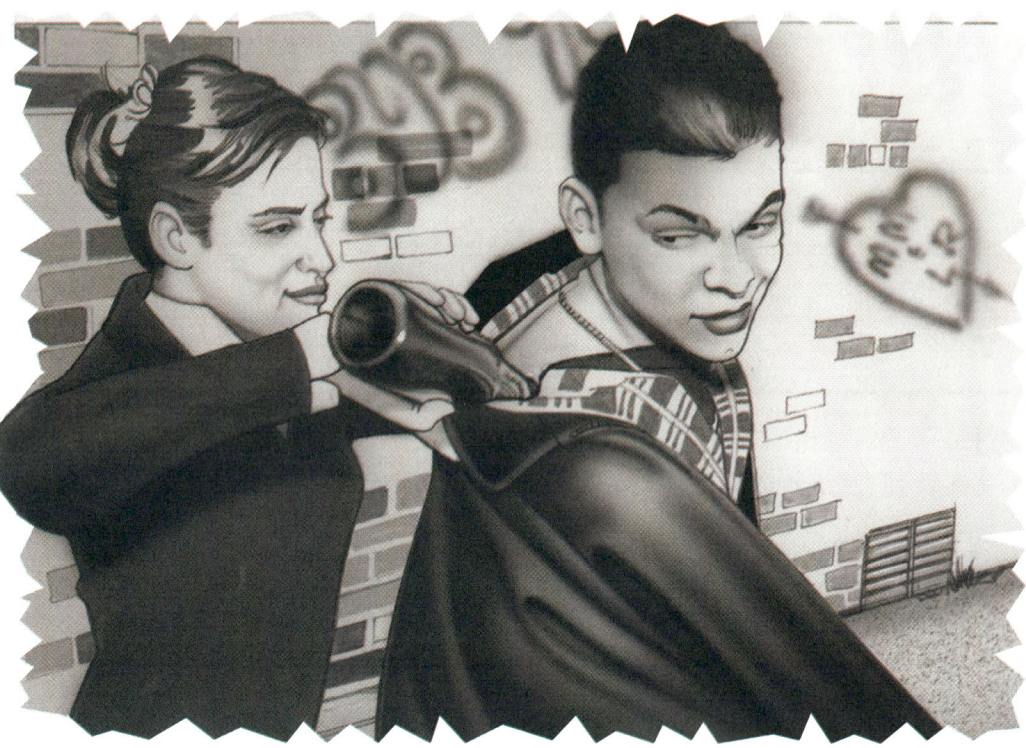

"This one's for you. You're going to need it because I won't be around."

It was Mike's first "No-Mores" meeting. He listened to the other kids' stories, trying to figure out how Amy had talked him into coming. Maybe he was crazy. Or maybe it was love….

Amy and Mike had been dating for six months. They were friends, too. They talked to each other easily about everything—well, maybe not everything. Amy hated his friends and she got really uptight when they drank. She had been after him again at the party, the night before the big game.

No Harm Done

"Come on Amy, don't start hassling me about having a few drinks." Mike made a face. He looked like a helpless puppy.

"I'm not hurting anyone." The guys erupted in laughter. Mike watched as Amy stiffened in anger. He knew he had to say something before she lost her cool. He reached out and put his arm around Amy's shoulder.

"Relax. I don't expect you to get wasted," he whispered softly in her ear. "Here, take a sip. This will calm you down."

"Listen Mike, every weekend it's like a six-pack is attached to your arm or something. All you do is drink. I'm beginning to wonder what means more to you, me or drinking with your buddies."

"Whoa! You know something, Amy, you're the

problem! You don't know how to relax."

To Mike's surprise, Amy apologized and asked for a drink.

"That's my girl," thought Mike. "She knows how to make a guy feel good in front of his friends."

Amy popped the cap off the bottle and placed one arm over Mike's shoulder.

"This one's for you," she said, pouring the liquid down his back. "You're going to need it because I won't be around."

Mike's friends roared in laughter. "Man, she really 'dissed' you!" Joe said.

"Come on Mike, no need to cry over spilled booze!" added Cory. The guys fell to the ground, rolling in laughter.

Mike was so stunned, he seemed unaware of his friends' jokes and their laughter. He left the party in a daze and headed home to change.

Anger Cools

The cool night air had a calming effect. He could still feel the effects of the alcohol, but his thoughts were clearer now. "Amy was right," he thought. "If I hadn't been drinking, I never would have treated her that way."

When he got home, Mike phoned Amy, but she wouldn't talk to him. "There's only one way to make her listen," he thought. "I'll have to apologize in person."

He walked over to Amy's apartment and knocked on the door. No one answered. The door was slightly open, Mike looked in; the living room was a wreck. In the center was Amy's mother sprawled across the couch, an empty bottle of wine lying on the carpet.

Now he understood Amy's concern. Drinking does affect more than just the drinker.

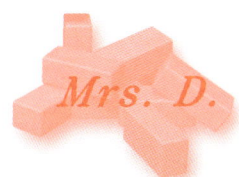

"STAND FIRM FOR WHAT IS RIGHT OR YOU WILL BE BENT BY THE WHIMS OF OTHERS."

Mrs. D.

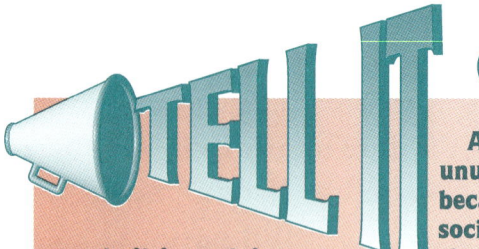

Accepted, Yet Risky

Alcohol is an unusual drug because society accepts it in certain situations. This acceptance makes it easier for drinking to become a problem for teens, families, and society.

Major Killer

Drinking comes with serious risks. Poor judgment caused by alcohol abuse results in highway accidents, homicides, assaults, on-the-job accidents, even rapes. Poor decisions due to the influence of alcohol can result in pregnancy and sexually transmitted diseases, including AIDS. Even unborn babies are affected when a pregnant woman drinks.

Billboards, movies, television, and sports advertising glamorize drinking. What is not shown is the one in ten Americans for whom it is a serious problem.

Levels of Dependence

Most people begin drinking in "social situations." They may drink at parties, before dinner, or perhaps to celebrate a special occasion. People who drink on occasion are called social drinkers.

Frequent drinking may turn the social drinker into a problem drinker. When alcohol is used to escape problems, to have fun, or to deal with stress, it has become a problem. The problem drinker often drinks alone.

A problem drinker runs the risk of becoming an alcoholic. Alcoholism is a disease that is physically and psychologically addicting. Alcohol becomes an important part of the person's daily life. The alcoholic's body changes; it needs alcohol to function. Going without alcohol causes withdrawal symptoms such as severe shaking, hallucinations, even death! Doctors feel that an alcoholic who successfully stops drinking must avoid alcohol for life.

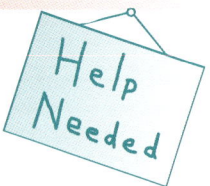

Alcoholics and their families usually need outside help, but until a problem is admitted, very little can be done. Alcohol abusers ready for help may turn to organizations such as **Alcoholics Anonymous (AA)**.

AA is an organization of recovering alcoholics who try to help others to stay alcohol-free. **Alateen** is a division of **AA** that helps teens who live with an alcoholic. **Al-anon**, also part of **AA**, helps family members cope while living with an alcoholic.

These groups teach that the alcoholic is responsible for his/her behavior. They encourage family members to avoid enabling behaviors.

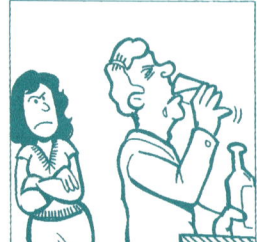
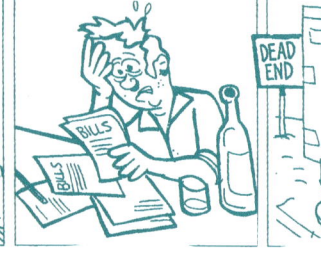
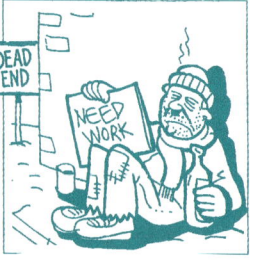

STREET SMART STRATEGIES

KNOWLEDGE POWER: Learn about the levels of alcohol dependence and the effects.
CORE VALUES: Depend upon yourself, not alcohol. Your behavior affects others.
PROACTION: Take a stand—attend a meeting of SADD, Alanon, or AA. Learn how they help.

BUZZ WORDS

1. **AA** — Alcoholics Anonymous, help group for alcoholics made up of alcoholics and recovered alcoholics
2. **Al-anon** — help group for family members affected by alcoholics
3. **Alateen** — help group for teens with alcoholic parents
4. **Alcoholic** — someone who is addicted to alcohol, whose body craves the drug
5. **Deny** — to pretend that a problem does not exist, make excuses, or blame someone else
6. **Enabling behaviors** — excuses made up by friends and families for the inappropriate actions of an alcoholic
7. **Gateway drug** — a drug that drug abusers may start with that leads to other drugs
8. **Glamorize** — to make something seem extremely attractive
9. **Hallucinations** — thoughts and fantasies that appear to be real
10. **Problem drinker** — someone who is dependent upon alcohol
11. **Rate of absorption** — time it takes for alcohol to get into your blood
12. **Social drinker** — someone who drinks with others on special occasions
12. **Impotence** — inability to have sex
12. **Sterility** — inability to have childre

ALCOHOL DEPENDENCE

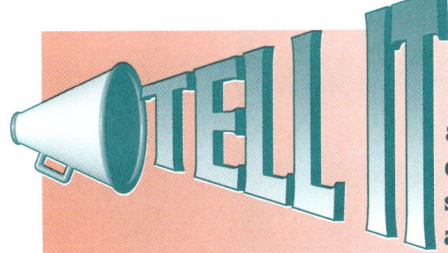

Risky Choices

Teenagers take chances with their lives when they drink. Poor decisions about sex, drugs, fighting or driving can change your life forever. Teenage drinkers are often encouraged by their friends to chug, or drink quickly. The smaller the person and the less the person weighs, the faster the alcohol will affect the body. The quicker alcohol is taken into the body, the more problems it causes since it is absorbed directly into the blood.

Combining alcohol with prescription drugs such as antihistamines is extremely dangerous. Taking non-prescription drugs or sleeping pills with alcohol can cause serious side effects: possibly coma, even death.

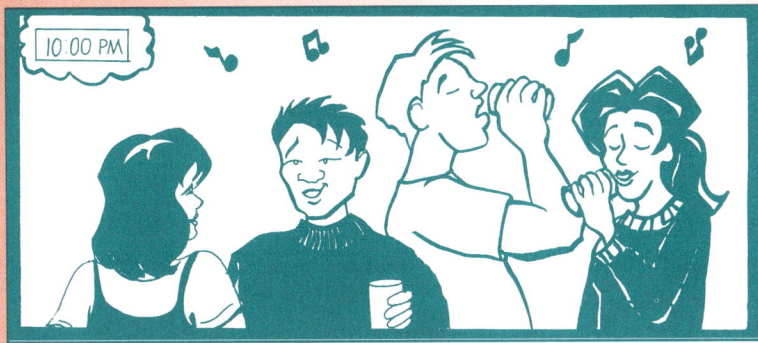
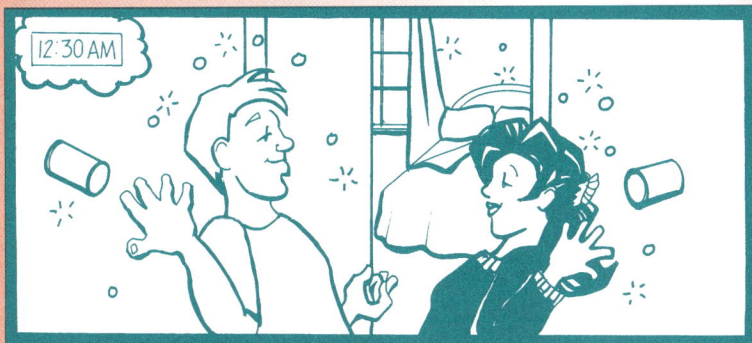
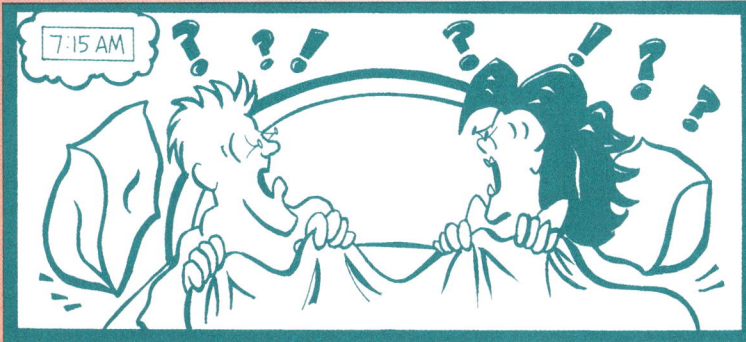
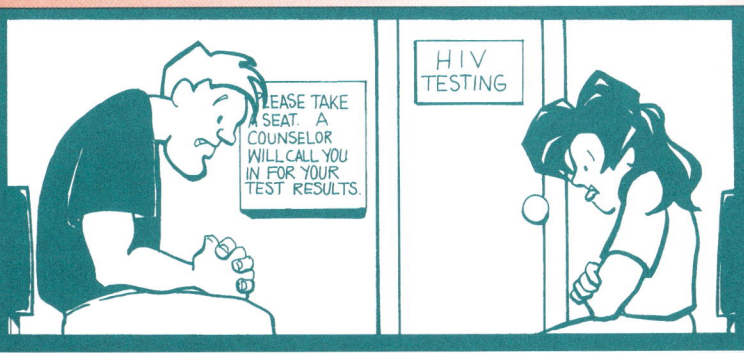

No Second Chance

The high rise in the number of teens infected with HIV/AIDS virus has caused many persons with AIDS to tell their stories. They encourage teens to abstain from alcohol. A great number of these people say they contracted AIDS as teenagers because they made poor decisions while under the influence of alcohol and do not have a second chance. They want all other teens to make decisions that will allow them to stay healthy.

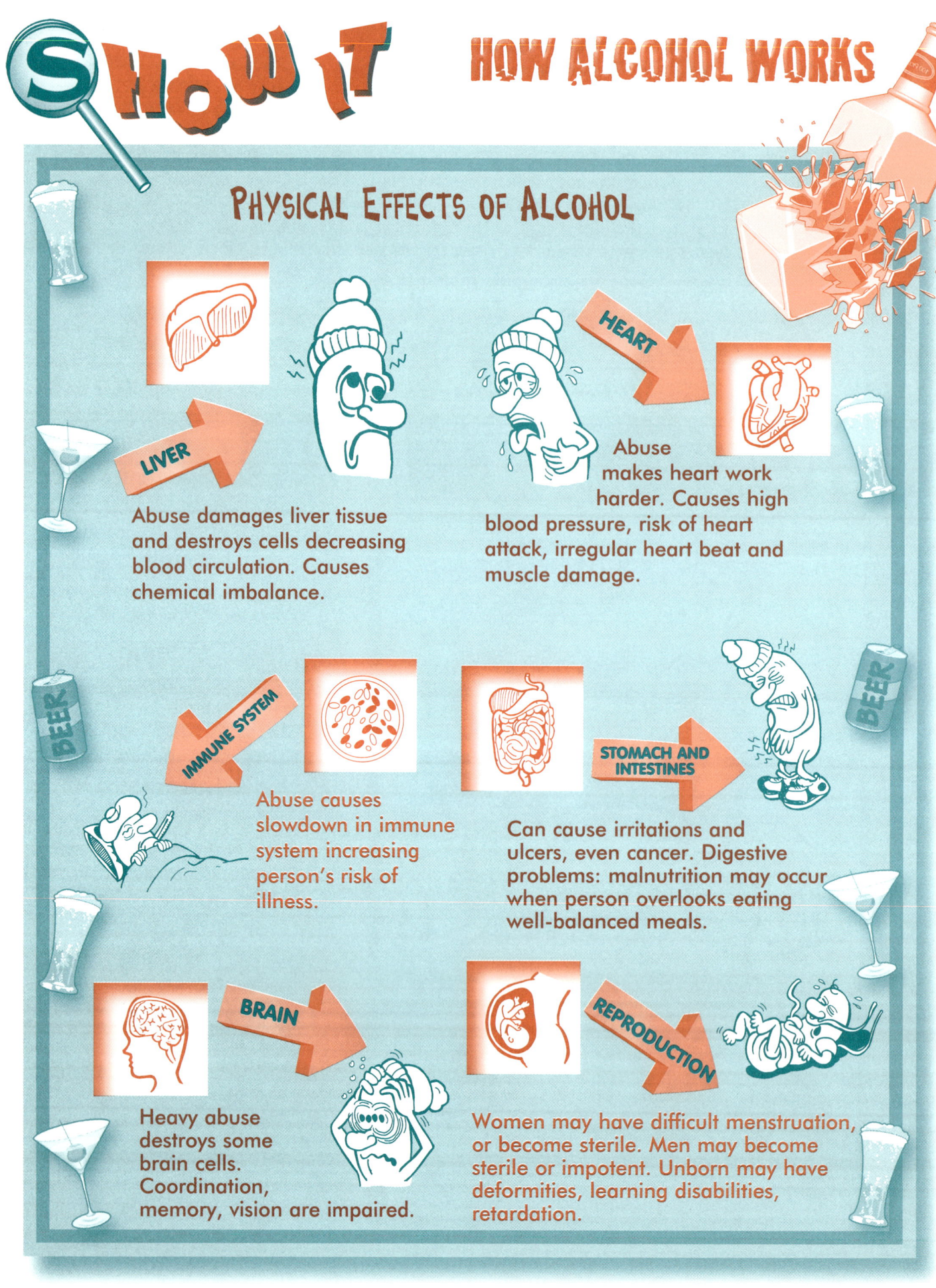

Show it

AVOID THESE ENABLING BEHAVIORS

☞ Lying or making excuses for irresponsible behaviors of the alcoholic ☞ Accepting their lies and excuses for irresponsible behaviors ☞ Covering up for them ☞ Giving them second and third chances for behaviors you know are not right

10 TIPS TO HELP THE ALCOHOLIC PROBLEM DRINKER

- Show you care by expressing your concern
- Be specific in telling them what things you have noticed or experienced that concern you
- Tell simply but honestly the feelings you have about their behaviors
- Try not to criticize them, focus on behaviors
- State your feelings positively and firmly, do not argue
- Offer your help and support, suggest going with them to get help
- Make a list of community, school, medical, religious experts who could help
- Try to get other friends or family members to support the effort for help
- Decide what you will do if the alcoholic repeats the behavior that concerns you
- If the alcoholic repeats the action that you want to stop, follow through on whatever you have said you will/will not do

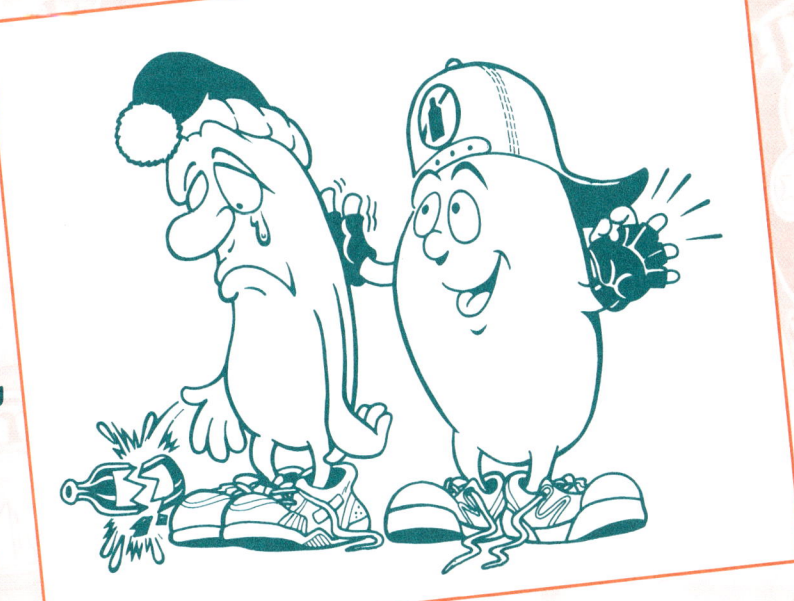

Are you a problem drinker? Answer and find out.

Yes   No

1. Do you drink to avoid problems?
2. Do you drink by yourself?
3. Do you hide the amount of drinking you do?
4. Do you "blackout" and forget what you've done?
5. Do you get into fights, arguments, or trouble when you drink?
6. Have you tried to stop but found you are unable to?
7. Do you drink in the morning?

(If you answer yes to even one of these questions, you have an alcohol problem.)

Reprinted Courtesy of National Council on Alcoholism and Drug Dependence, Inc.

HOOK, LINE, AND SINKER

HOOK: The drugs that get people hooked. **LINE:** The lie that gets them to take the drugs. **SINKER:** The bad results of taking drugs.

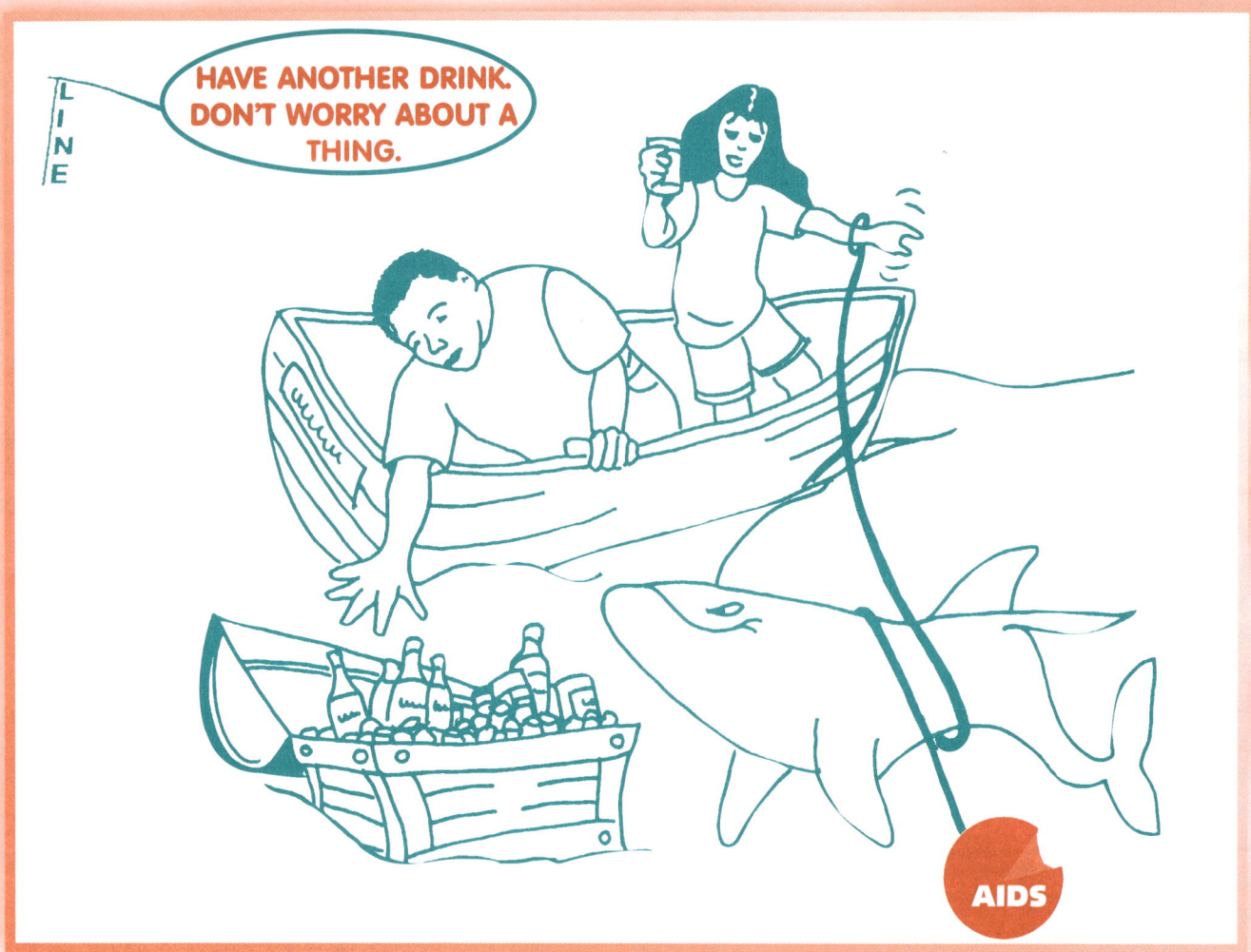

THINK ABOUT IT...

Use the cartoon above to answer the following questions:

Name the drug the boaters are abusing.
_____
_____

What line is being used to convince the girl to drink?
_____
_____

What disease are the boaters at risk for while under the influence of alcohol?
_____
_____

Be Street Smart

Support, but don't enable. Contact support groups for help.

For Advice And Information Call:
Al-Anon/Alateen Family Group
Information Line
1-800-344-2666

26   ALCOHOL DEPENDENCE   Street Smarts

CHECKUP

MATCHING

Column A | Column B

1. ___ social drinking
2. ___ Alateen
3. ___ alcoholism
4. ___ AA

a. organization to help teens who live with an alcoholic
b. Alcoholics Anonymous
c. "light" drinking at social events
d. disease in which body needs alcohol to function

MULTIPLE CHOICE

1. **Which is an enabling behavior?**
   a. Going to Al-Anon
   b. Joining SADD
   c. Making excuses when someone is drunk

2. **Problem drinkers**
   a. are easy to recognize
   b. absorb alcohol faster
   c. can be helped

3. **Alcohol**
   a. is okay for teen
   b. is a gateway drug
   c. helps solve problems

4. **Alcohol is absorbed faster**
   a. on an empty stomach
   b. if you drink slowly
   c. if you sit down while drinking

FILL IN THE BLANKS

encourage   unusual   Al-anon
levels of dependence   alcoholic

Alcohol is an _____ drug since society accepts it in certain situations but not in others. Advertisers sometimes _____ people to drink. People go through _____ when it comes to abusing alcohol. If a person depends upon alcohol to function, they are considered an _____. One group that can help the families of alcoholics is called _____.

TAKE A STAND

Dear Mrs. D.

IMPROVE YOUR REFUSAL SKILLS

Dear Mrs. D.:

Dad manages a business. With times so bad, he has had to lay off many employees. He has had to go into debt to pay bills.

Instead of two cocktails when he gets home from work, he drinks until he falls asleep. He is so hung over in the morning that he sometimes doesn't go into work until noon.

People from work call wanting to know where he is. He tells us to say that he is out of town at a conference.

I'm scared of what he is doing to himself. What can I do?

Signed,
Tired of Lying

Write how you would answer if you were Mrs. D.

Mrs. D. Answers:
_____
_____
_____
_____
_____
_____
_____
_____
_____
_____

Show that you recognize the danger by completing the exercise below.

George, a senior in high school, has been working part-time as a bus boy at a restaurant. Most of the other bus boys go to the local college. Lately, George has been hanging out with them. George likes being with the older guys, but lately has been feeling left out because he doesn't drink. Furthermore, when he tries to discourage them from drinking and driving, they tell him to "get with the program."

1. <u>Underline</u> a sentence that shows how George's job is putting him at risk for alcohol abuse.

2. (Circle) a sentence that shows how George's new friends are pressuring him.

3. **LIST** what George could do to make his college buddies respect his no-drinking decision.
_____
_____

Write the "coolest" way to say, "No!"

1. **The Offer** Your cousin, a heavy weekend drinker, invites you to an important party.

   You say _____
   _____

2. **The Dare** "Your crowd goes to a local hangout. Your best friend says, "I bet I can finish two drinks before you."

   You say _____
   _____

   BACK OFF

3. **The Threat** Your date says, "You better not just drink soda tonight. I'm tired of your goody-goody act."

   You say _____
   _____

4. **The Feel Good Approach** "I know that you are down about not making the team. A drink will help you forget."

   You say _____
   _____

28   ALCOHOL DEPENDENCE   Street Smarts

YOUR TURN

SPEAK OUT

1. How can the sale of alcoholic beverages to teens be more strictly enforced?

_____
_____

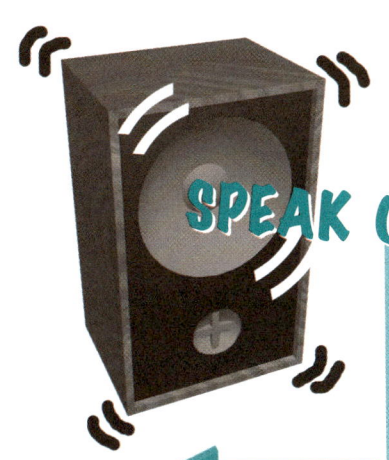

2. Unborn babies are affected by the alcohol use of the mother. Deformities, retardation, and learning disabilities may result. What should society do to protect unborn babies?

_____
_____

ASK A PARENT AN ADULT GUARDIAN

ASK: When you were growing up, did you have any family members who had a serious drinking problem? How did the family handle it? What advice would you give teens about drinking?

LIGHTS, CAMERA, ACTION!

Setting: You are the editor of your school newspaper. You have the responsibility of making sure that your reporters give fair coverage to issues. Last weekend, three top basketball players were suspended from the team for the rest of the year because they were caught drinking. Playoffs are coming up.

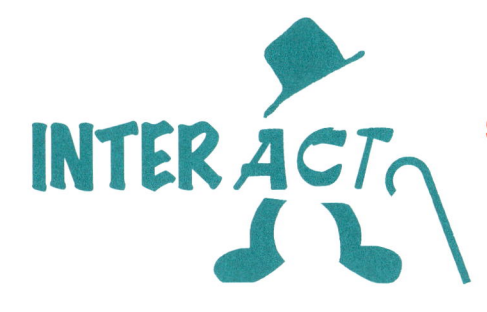

Situation: You must report the incident since it affects the student body.

Solution: Act out your discussion of coverage with your staff. Suggest some ways that the paper could make this negative action a positive action.

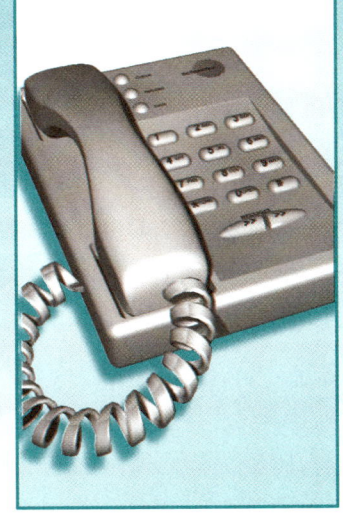

INTERACT

Teen Talk

1. Your best friend moves out of state. She invites you to visit. You accept, but during your visit you discover that the only thing your friend likes to do is get drunk. She calls it "partying". You tell her that what she's doing is more than partying. She tells you to "Mind your own business." What do you do next?

2. List some concerns that Amy must overcome to make a responsible decision.

THE PEOPLES PUBLISHING GROUP, 1-800-822-1080. COPYING PROHIBITED BY LAW.

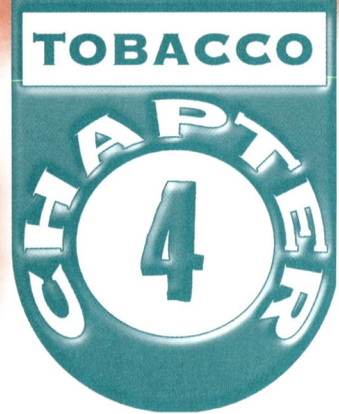

TOBACCO
CHAPTER 4
GOING UP IN SMOKE

Sergeant Leguero opened the door and immediately sensed that something was wrong! Smoke was coming from beneath the door of the storeroom where the "No-Mores" met each week. He ran to the door and felt for heat.

"Is anyone in there?" he yelled, yanking the door open.

Twelve voices shouted, "Surprise!"

On the table was a heart-shaped cake with twenty burning cigarettes for candles. The white icing was stained brown from the smoke and covered with ashes. Mrs. D. touched Leguero's shoulder gently in a silent show of support for what was coming next.

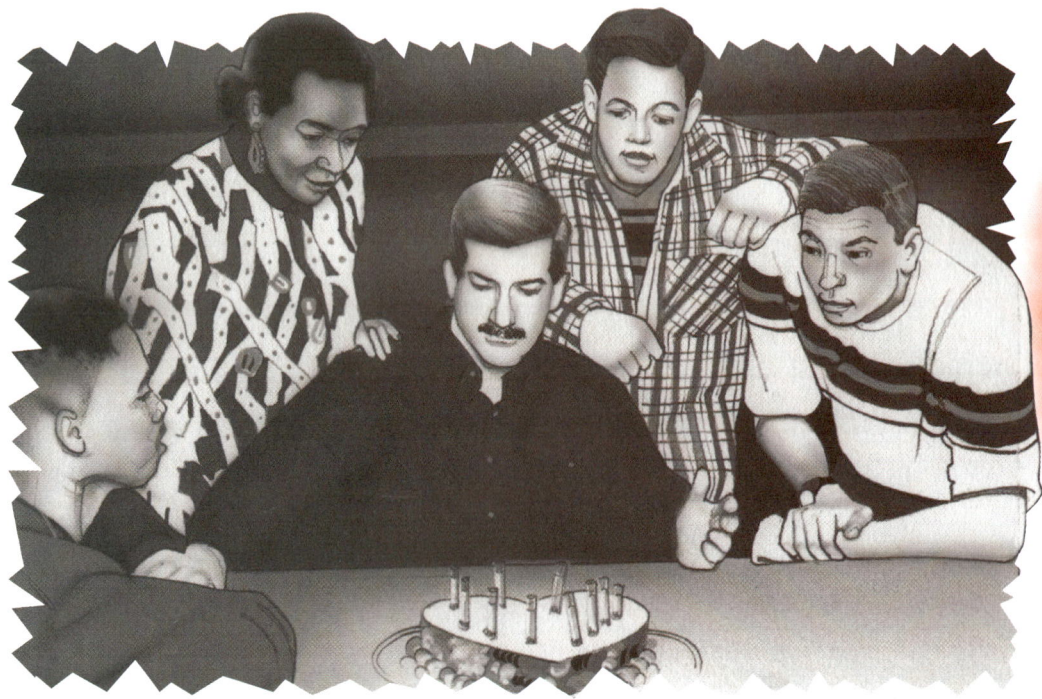

"You can't be naggin' us all the time about druggin' when you smoke..."

Mixed Feelings

Leguero wiped his face. He felt a mixture of relief, surprise, and a small knot of anger that he was trying to hide.

"It's hard to believe you made it to fifty with kids like us on the streets, especially with all those cigarette butts you're smoking," George joked.

"Yeah, well, you kids drove me to it!" Leguero teased. He was the first to admit that the "No-Mores" weren't the real reason behind the habit he knew he had to quit. No need to tell them that he hadn't had a cigarette for years until his wife left him.

"What's with the cigarette cake?" he asked, puzzled.

30　　　　　TOBACCO　　　　　Street Smarts

George took the lead. "What do you think, Lego? You can't be naggin' us all the time about druggin' when you smoke over a pack a day. We decided it was your turn to take the heat. Face it, Lego, you're not anywhere near the shape you were in before you started smoking again."

Leguero said nothing. He knew they were right.

Mrs. D. brought out the real cake and placed it on the table. It was shaped like a cigarette box with a big X drawn through it.

Kisha handed him a beautifully wrapped gift. It was heavy.

Three Ways To Quit

Leguero read the card out loud: "Three ways to quit." He slowly opened the box and pulled out his gifts.

First, he found a small package. Inside the box were two individually wrapped, oval adhesive patches, each labelled 'NICOTINE PATCH.' He quickly read the directions about the patch. Each week, he was to peel off the backing and place one on his skin, much like a band aid. He saw that each patch could be easily removed at the end of a week and replaced by a fresh one.

Next, he unwrapped a gold medallion with a note on it. "If the patch doesn't work, take this to a hypnotist." Leguero smiled.

The last item in the box was a frozen turkey. Lequero got the point. He would go cold turkey starting now!

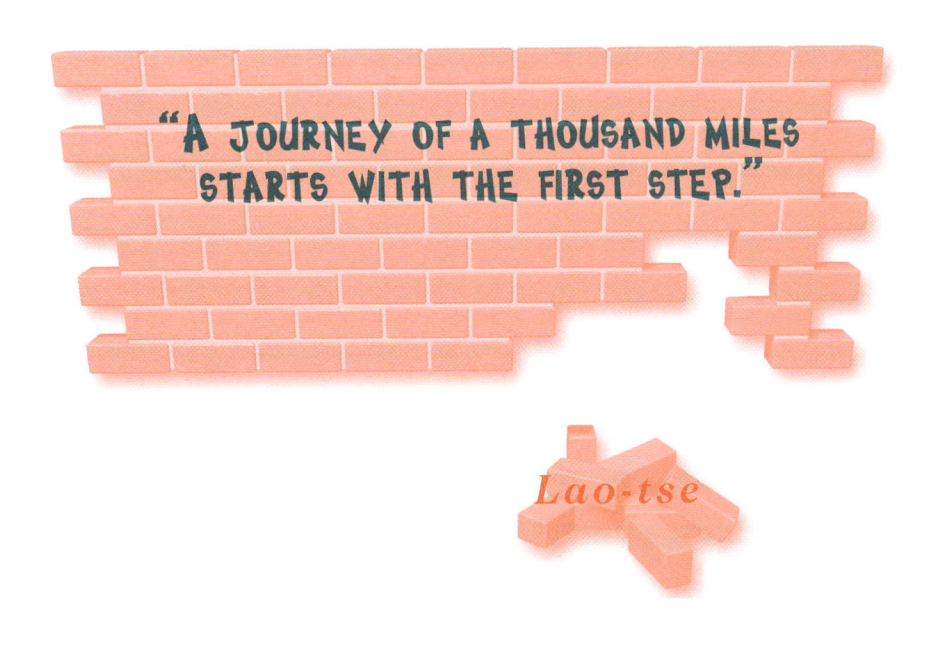

"A JOURNEY OF A THOUSAND MILES STARTS WITH THE FIRST STEP."

Lao-tse

TELL IT

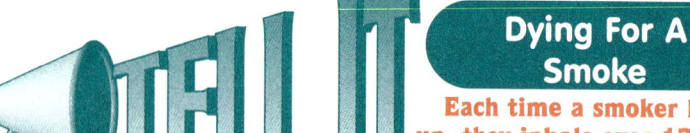

Dying For A Smoke

Each time a smoker lights up, they inhale over 1200 chemicals. Here are a few: **Carbon monoxide** is a colorless, odorless gas, perhaps the worst poison in tobacco smoke. When a smoker **inhales**, **carbon monoxide** passes into the lungs and enters the bloodstream. The person can't get the oxygen he/she needs. The **carbon monoxide** produces dizziness and then damages cells when oxygen is replaced by **carbon monoxide**.

Tar is a dark sticky substance that clings to fingers, teeth, throat and lungs. It makes breathing difficult. It stains teeth and fingers. **Nicotine** causes tobacco addiction. It speeds up the heart rate and slows down the flow of blood to hands and feet. It also causes a "nicotine fit" when a person tries to quit smoking.

Scientists have also proven that some of the chemicals **inhaled** while smoking are **carcinogenic**, they cause cancer. Research has shown that lung cancer, bladder cancer, pancreatic cancer, and cancer of the mouth can all be linked to smoking or **chewing tobacco**.

Passive Smoking

Sadly, smokers are not the only one affected by the dangers of tobacco abuse. As a smoker **inhales**, some of the poisons are released into the air that non-smokers breathe. Non-smokers breathe this **side-stream** or secondhand smoke into their lungs. Then, they too have an increased chance of developing cancer.

To protect non-smokers, laws have been passed to limit areas where people can smoke. It is illegal to smoke in any enclosed public place.

The Truth About Smoking

Smoking endangers your health and the health of people around you. Persons with respiratory problems such as asthma are particularly at risk. Persons who smoke have bad breath, smoke odor on their clothing, and brown stains on their teeth and clothes.

Worse, the U.S. Center for Disease Control reports that tobacco kills about 400,000 Americans each year, almost ten times the number killed by car accidents!

STREET SMART STRATEGIES

KNOWLEDGE POWER: Learn about the dangers of tobacco use.

CORE VALUES: Develop self-discipline. Don't smoke.

PROACTION: Take a stand—practice tobacco refusal skills.

BUZZ WORDS

1. **Aversion therapy** — makes smoking unpleasant so smokers avoid smoking
2. **Carbon monoxide** — a colorless, odorless, poisonous gas that replaces oxygen in the lungs
3. **Carcinogenic** — cancer causing
4. **Chewing tobacco** — tobacco placed between the gums and teeth and chewed
5. **Cold turkey** — method of quitting smoking by just stopping
6. **Hypnosis** — method of quitting smoking using the power of suggestion
7. **Inhale** — breathe into lungs
8. **Nicotine** — a chemical that causes the desire for tobacco
9. **Nicotine fit** — addicted person's body demands nicotine, person feels like they must have tobacco
10. **Passive smoking** — non-smoker breathes in smoke of smoker
11. **Side-stream smoke** — secondhand smoke; smoke-filled air around a smoker
12. **Smokeless tobacco** — tobacco sniffed, chewed or held in mouth, but not smoked
13. **Snuff** — finely ground tobacco sniffed through nostrils or held against gums

Show It

WHAT ABOUT SMOKELESS TOBACCO?

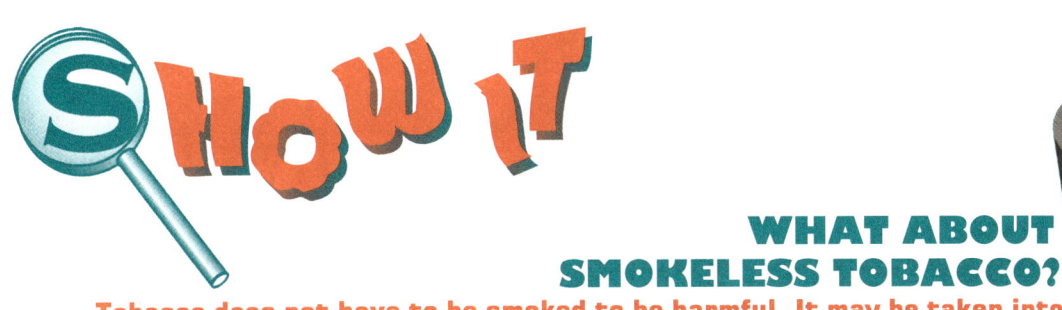

Tobacco does not have to be smoked to be harmful. It may be taken into the mouth as chewing tobacco. It may be inhaled through the nose or held between the cheek and gums as snuff. Nicotine can enter the body through the nose or mouth and greatly increases the risk for nose, mouth, or throat cancer.

Most people who smoke, chew or sniff tobacco report that they started at a young age. They "hung out" with friends who used tobacco. They thought it made them look older. They felt they were part of "the group." Most believed that they could quit whenever they wanted.

With each cigarette, "chew", or "sniff" nicotine gradually changes the chemistry of the body. Soon it causes a craving which leads to addiction.

THE GOOD NEWS

There is good news. The good news is that when a smoker quits, positive things begin to happen. Many of the harmful effects of tobacco are reduced. Since 1964 when the U.S. Surgeon General warned the American public about the dangers of smoking, more than 30 million Americans have quit.

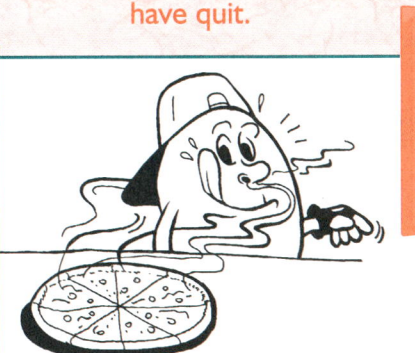

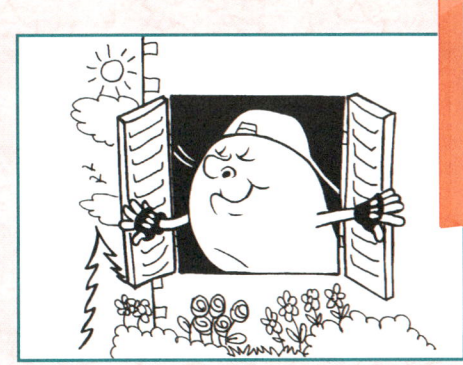

TIME AFTER QUITTING: 1 Day
CHANGES IN BODY: Oxygen level returns to normal. Chance of heart attack is reduced.

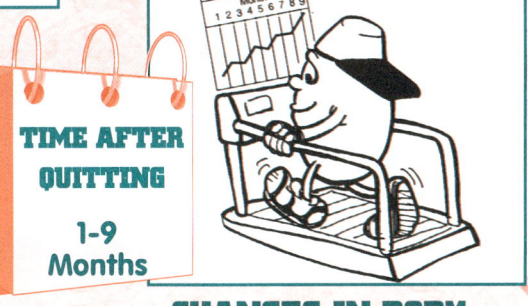

TIME AFTER QUITTING: 2nd or 3rd Week
CHANGES IN BODY: Sense of smell and taste improve.

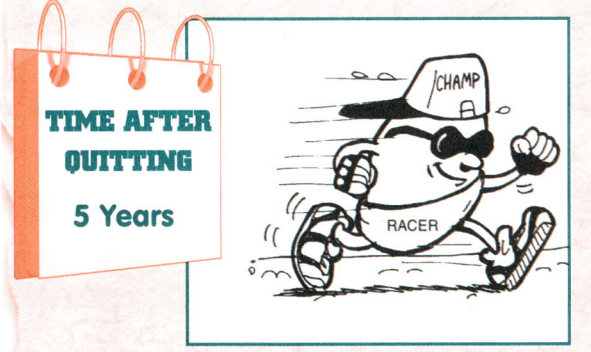

TIME AFTER QUITTING: 1-9 Months
CHANGES IN BODY: Circulation, lung functions, energy, improve. Risk of infection reduced.

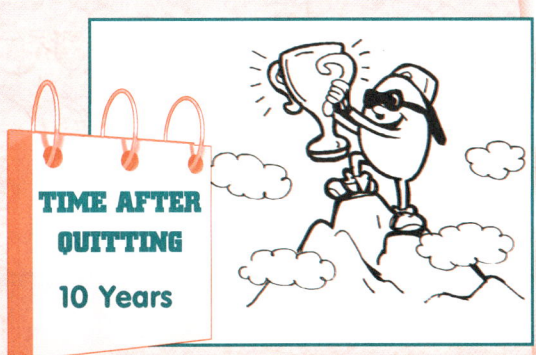

TIME AFTER QUITTING: 5 Years
CHANGES IN BODY: Risk of lung cancer, heart disease, is greatly reduced.

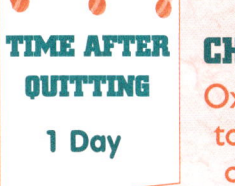

TIME AFTER QUITTING: 10 Years
CHANGES IN BODY: Pre-cancerous cells are replaced by the body. Risk of cancer almost equal to that of life-time non-smoker.

SHOW IT

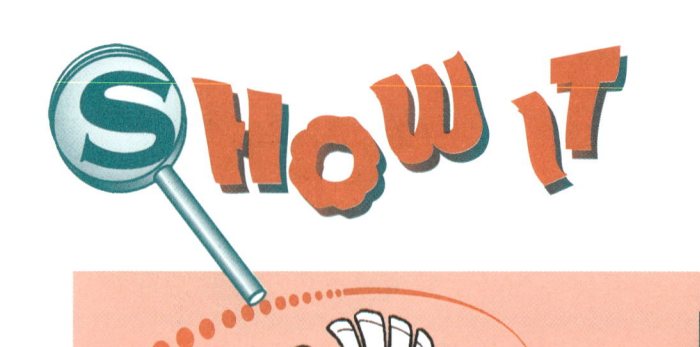

5 WAYS TO QUIT

COLD TURKEY

WHAT IT MEANS	Quit immediately, 100%
PROS	Gets nicotine out of body quickly
CONS	Difficult to do

PART/TIME

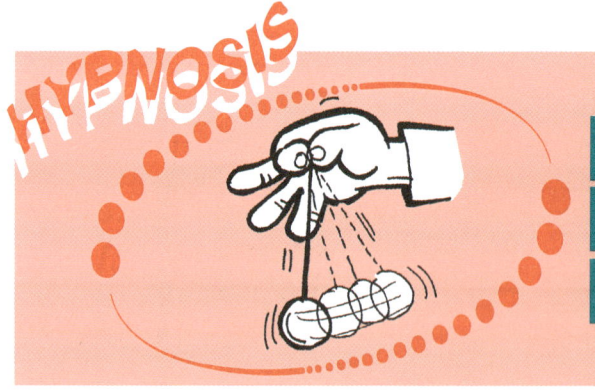

WHAT IT MEANS	Quit gradually; switch to low tar nicotine cigarettes
PROS	Easier for body to adjust
CONS	Never finish nicotine with-drawal

HYPNOSIS

WHAT IT MEANS	Hypnotist uses power of suggestion
PROS	Can be easy if person is willing
CONS	Expensive, and not always effective

AVERSION

WHAT IT MEANS	Make smoking distasteful (e.g. force person to breathe stale smoke)
PROS	Makes smoking unpleasant
CONS	Unreliable results

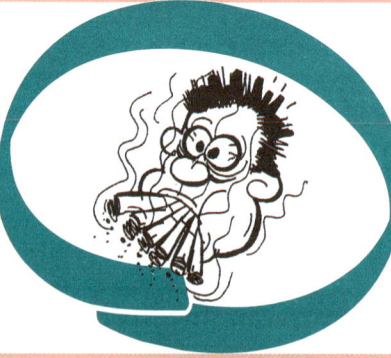

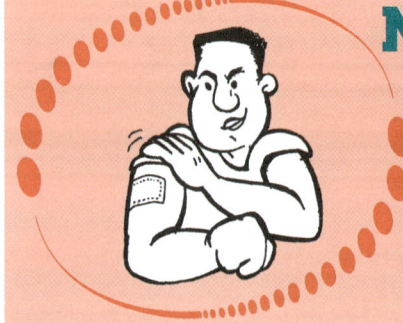

MEDICAL PRODUCTS

WHAT IT MEANS	Tablets, patches, nicotine gum work by regulating desire for nicotine
PROS	Provides daily assistance
CONS	May need doctor's care; expensive; can cause side effects; leaves nicotine dependence untreated

TOBACCO — Street Smarts

HOOK, LINE, AND SINKER

HOOK: The drugs that get people hooked. **LINE:** The lie that gets them to take the drugs. **SINKER:** The bad results of taking drugs.

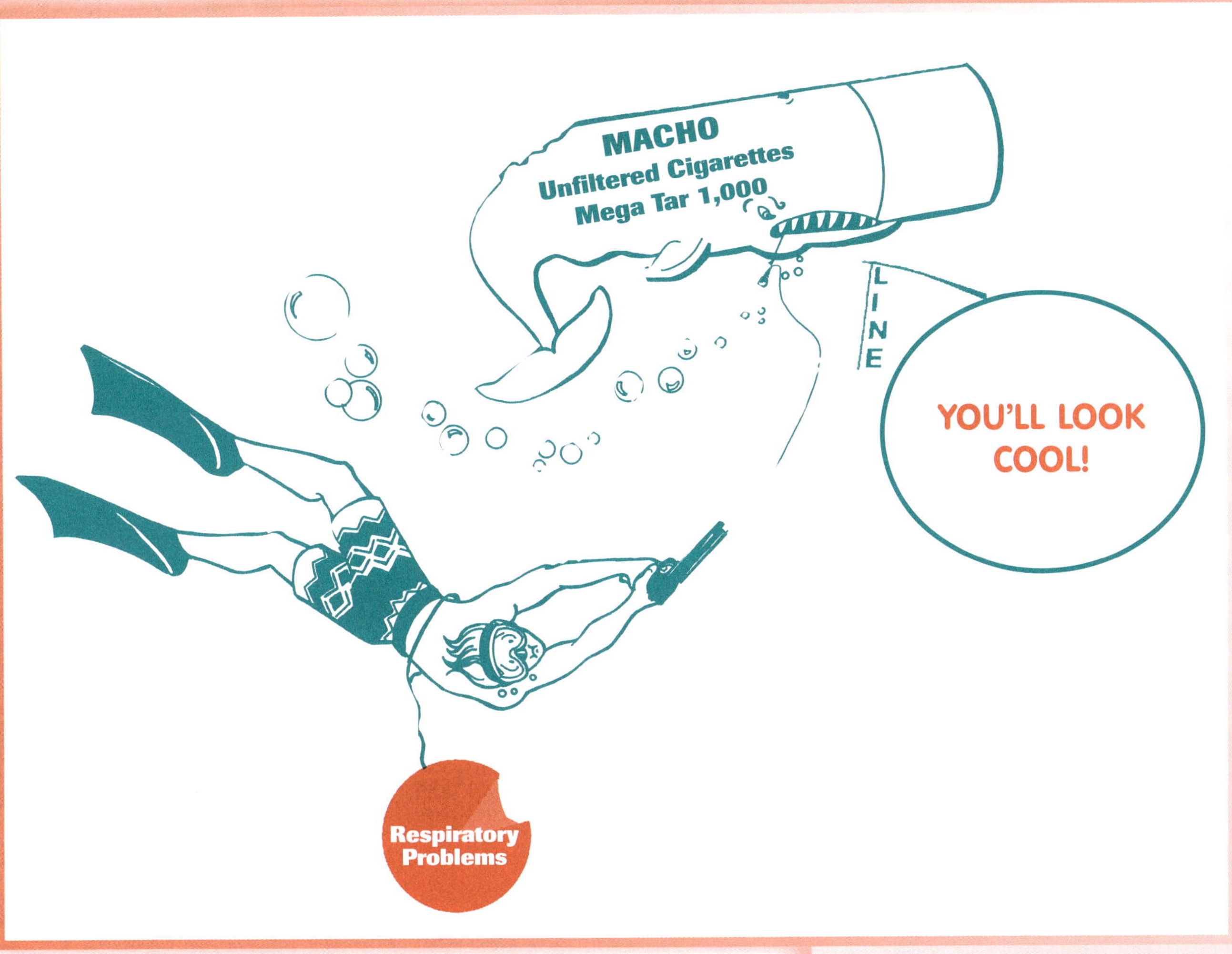

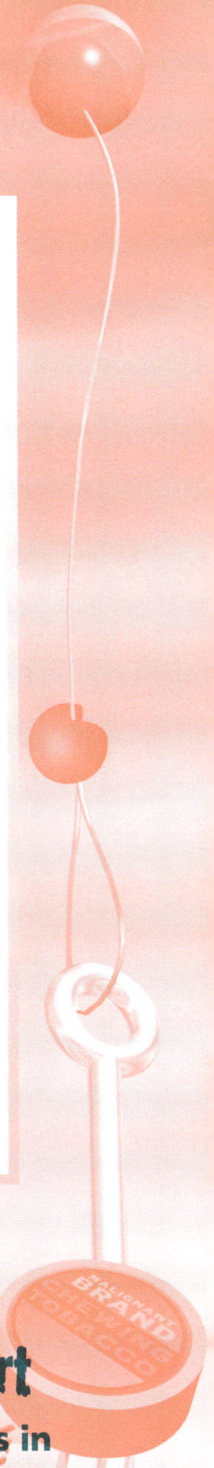

[Cartoon: A swimmer reaches for a cigarette labeled "MACHO Unfiltered Cigarettes Mega Tar 1,000". A speech bubble (LINE) says "YOU'LL LOOK COOL!" A red circle labeled "Respiratory Problems" appears below.]

THINK AB💡UT IT...

Use the cartoon above to answer the following questions:

HOOK — On what drug is this swimmer hooked?
_____
_____

LINE — What is Macho telling the swimmer?
_____
_____

SINKER — What problem for the swimmer can continued abuse cause?
_____
_____

Be Street Smart

Deal with smokers in a positive and affirmative manner. Help yourself and others to stay tobacco-free!

For Advice and Information Call:

1-800-784-7357
American Cancer Society Information Help Line

THE PEOPLES PUBLISHING GROUP, 1-800-822-1080. COPYING PROHIBITED BY LAW.

CHECKUP

MATCHING

Column A	Column B
1. ___ snuff	a. to breathe into lungs
2. ___ inhale	b. smokeless tobacco
3. ___ carcinogen	c. causes addiction to tobacco
4. ___ nicotine	d. cancer causing
5. ___ side-stream smoke	e. smoke surrounding smoker

FILL IN THE BLANKS

desire   habit   heal   cancer   1200   hazardous   quit   chemicals

Smoking is a _____. The Surgeon General stated that smoking is _____ to your health. When a person smokes, he or she breathes in over _____ poisonous _____. Some of these poisons can cause _____.

Because of the dangers of smoking, over 30 million Americans have _____. Once a person has quit, the body begins to _____. The key to quitting is a strong _____.

MULTIPLE CHOICE

1. **A form of tobacco that is sniffed**
   a. cigarette
   b. snuff
   c. chewing tobacco

2. **The chemical in tobacco that causes addiction**
   a. tar
   b. carbon monoxide
   c. nicotine

3. **Cold turkey is a method of quitting smoking by**
   a. stopping completely
   b. hypnosis
   c. using the patch

4. **The chemical that stains teeth and fingers**
   a. tar
   b. nicotine
   c. carbon monoxide

5. **Smoking in an enclosed, public place is**
   a. legal
   b. illegal
   c. allowed

TOBACCO   Street Smarts

TAKE A STAND

Dear Mrs. D.

IMPROVE YOUR REFUSAL SKILLS

Dear Mrs. D.:

I've been smoking for three years. I know it's not good for me, but my friends all smoke. We have always made fun of the "health-nuts" who don't smoke.

My new boyfriend tells me my breath stinks and so do my clothes and my hair. He doesn't think there is anything attractive about a girl who smokes. I'm beginning to agree.

I want to quit, but I want to keep my same friends. How can I do it?

Signed,
Smoking Sally

Write how you would answer if you were Mrs. D.

Mrs. D. Answers:
_____
_____
_____
_____
_____
_____
_____
_____
_____

Show that you recognize the danger by completing the exercise below.

Sue thought it would be fun to stay over at the White's home. She really likes Jenny and her family. The four older brothers, their father, mother and Jenny all have so much fun talking over dinner, sometimes it takes hours to finish a meal.

Everyone in Jenny's family, except Jenny, smokes. Smoking seems to go with talking, with coffee, with dessert, with phone calls, with everything. Even though Mrs. White is pregnant, she smokes like a chimney.

1. <u>Underline</u> a sentence that shows why Sue likes visiting the White family.

2. (Circle) two sentences that show how Jenny might be at risk for becoming a problem smoker.

3. Sue dislikes the smoke. How can she handle the situation without being rude?
_____
_____

Write the coolest way to say, "No!"

1. **The Offer** "Hey, someone left these butts on the counter. Let's have one."
   You say: _____
   _____
   _____

2. **The Dare** "Yo, José, are you too chicken to try a cigarette?"
   You say: _____
   _____
   _____

   BACK OFF

3. **The Threat** "Look Marissa, if you're not going to have a few smokes with us, I'm going to tell everyone that you're a nerd."
   You say: _____
   _____
   _____

4. **The Feel Good Approach** "The girls will think you're more grown up. You'll feel better talking to them."
   You say: _____
   _____

YOUR TURN

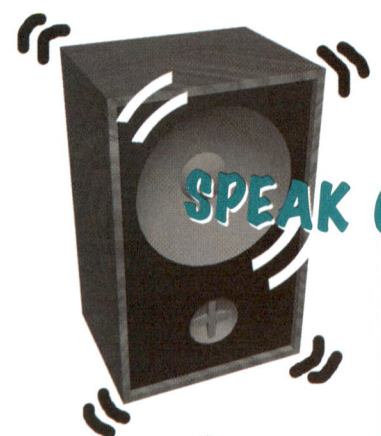

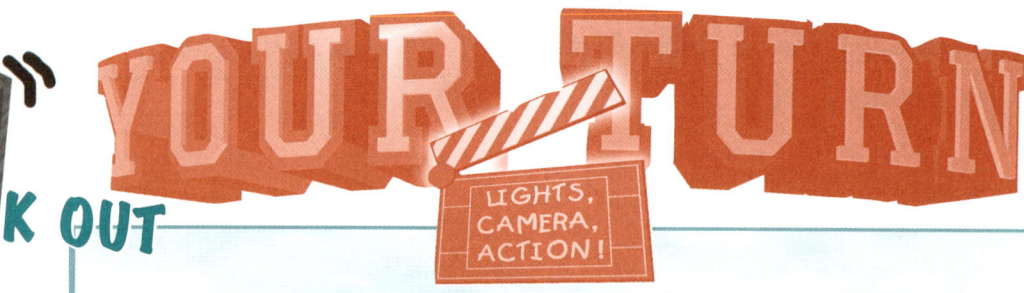

SPEAK OUT

1 Should cigar smokers be treated differently than cigarette smokers? If so, why? How? If not, why?

_____
_____

2 List two things you could do to help a family member or friend who is trying to quit smoking.

_____
_____

ASK A PARENT AN ADULT GUARDIAN

When you were growing up what reasons did kids give for smoking? List the reasons. Are the reasons the same as today?

INTERACT

Setting: You are the principal of a Jr. High School. On your way home from work you notice that a growing number of students are hanging out by the candy store smoking.

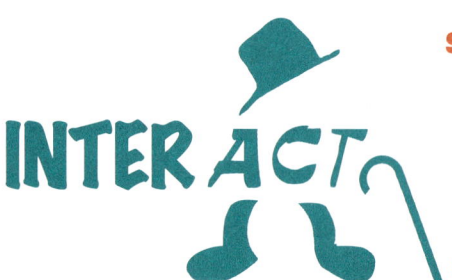

Situation: One of the students, Walter, is much respected by all the others. He is a young man who "thinks for himself". If Walter quits, you feel that it would encourage many of the others to quit. You decide to meet with Walter to see if you can get him to quit.

Solution: Act out the scene between you and Walter.

Teen Talk

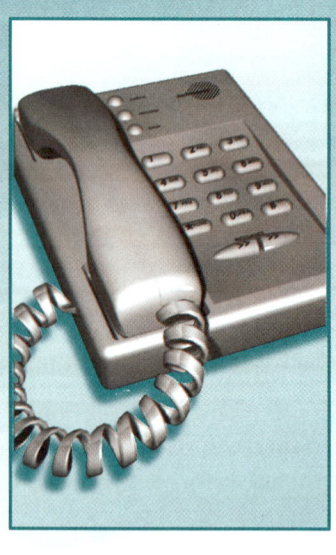

1. You take your girlfriend out for Valentine's Day to a nice restaurant. She asks to sit in the non-smoking section. The man at the next table lights up a cigar. How do you handle the situation?

2. You finally buy the car you have been working so hard to get. You have a "thing" about keeping it looking and smelling good. A friend asks you for a ride home. On the way, he pulls out a cigarette and starts to light up. What do you do?

TOBACCO — Street Smarts

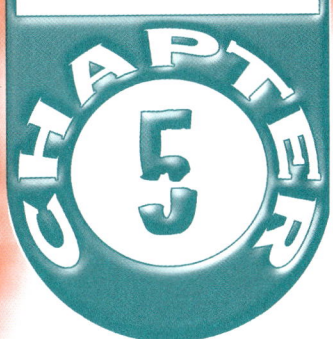

MARIJUANA
CHAPTER 5
"THE BURN OUT"

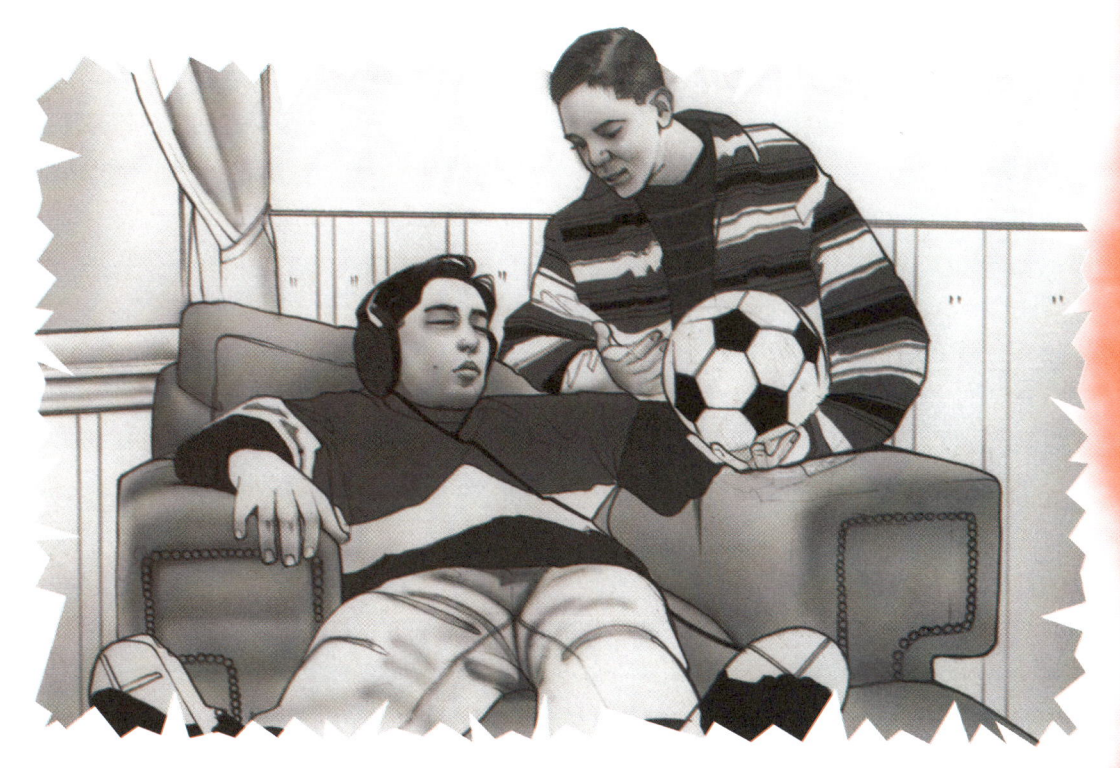

"...NO PRESSURES, NO WORRIES, NO THOUGHTS ABOUT SOCCER OR SCHOOL..."

Mrs. D. wondered if Frankie would volunteer to speak tonight. The "No-Mores" had nicknamed him, "The Burnout." They all knew he smoked a lot of pot. What they didn't know was why. Mrs. D. dismissed the idea. Maybe it's too soon, she thought, but to her surprise, Frankie began to speak.

"I guess I was bored. My best friend, Jamie, had gone to soccer camp for the summer, but I had no money to go. So, I was just kind of hanging out, not doing much of anything. Well, one day on the way home from the mall, I noticed a bunch of guys on the bus laughing and acting kind of stupid. I recognized one of the guys in the group from school. His name was Charles and he recognized me too. He came over and asked me if I liked to 'party'. I didn't want to sound stupid so I said, 'Sure'."

Mistake

"That was my first mistake. But at the time, I didn't know it. Charles invited me to 'party' with the group. He said I'd get to meet some girls. I jumped at the chance even though I wasn't too comfortable around girls.

"When I got to the party, everyone was stoned. Beer cans were all over the floor and the air was thick with weed. I'm barely in the door when this really cute girl comes up to me, giggling. Next thing I know she puts her arms around me and holds a joint to my lips. I mean, what could I do?"

"One thing led to another and before long I was 'partying' all the time. I felt cool. There was no pressure, no worries, no thoughts about soccer or school until Jamie came home. He was all psyched up about us both making the Varsity soccer team. He wanted to teach me all the soccer moves he had learned."

"I wasn't interested; soccer didn't matter to me anymore. It was fine for Jamie, but I had new friends, they didn't care about sports. By the time the summer was over, I was getting high every day. My eyes were always bloodshot."

"Mom didn't suspect that I was smoking pot at first. She was busy with her new boyfriend and basically left me alone, trusting me not to get into trouble. But then a few months ago, Mom started asking all kinds of questions. She wanted to know why I wasn't hanging out with Jamie anymore and why I wasn't playing soccer."

"You must have had a run in with with the cops to be here," said Kevin. "What happened?"

"You could say it was the school's fault for having open lunch periods! See, our school is really too crowded to have everyone eat lunch in the cafeteria. Most of us go to the park or to the deli to eat. Hey, with nobody watching, it seemed like a great time to smoke a joint and mellow out before the afternoon classes."

Dealing

"Then I had this really great idea to make some money. The kids were always asking to share my stuff, why didn't I sell it to them? So I had this reefer business going at lunch time in the park right across from the school. It was convenient. Business was great, and so was the money."

"Did you notice I said, '*was great*?' That's because I thought I was so clever, I never noticed that I was being watched. Then one day in English class, the principal called me into his office. The police were waiting there for me. They handcuffed me and read me my rights. And that was the end of my business and my life as I knew it."

"Wait a minute," Leguero cut in. "Which life do you miss? The life before pot or those months after you started smoking pot?"

"YOU START THE JOURNEY TO THE TOP THE DAY THAT YOU STOP MAKING EXCUSES AND BEGIN TAKING RESPONSIBILITY FOR YOURSELF."

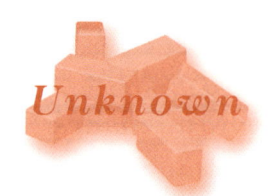

Unknown

TELL IT

The Pot Plant

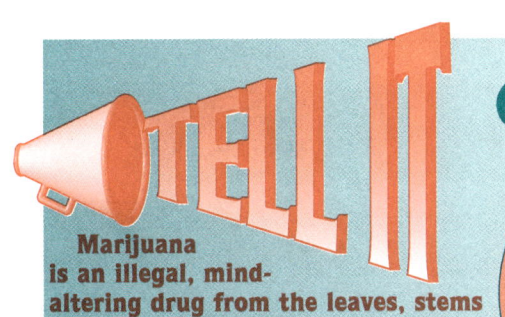

Marijuana is an illegal, mind-altering drug from the leaves, stems and flowers of the cannabis sativa plant. The drug goes by many names: weed, chronic, pot, reefer, grass. The main mind-altering chemical it contains is tetrahydrocannabinol, or THC.

All marijuana is not the same strength. Different forms of the cannabis plant have different amounts of THC. The strength of marijuana is determined by the type of plant, where it is grown, when it is harvested, and what part of the plant is used.

The most common form of pot comes from the dried flowers, stems, and leaves of the plant. Hash or hashish comes from the resin of leaves and flowers. It usually contains five to ten times more THC than common pot. Hash oil contains up to fifty percent THC and is the most powerful form of the drug.

The stronger the marijuana, the more serious the effects on the user.

How Is It Used?

The dried leaves, buds or flowers can be smoked in cigarette form called a joint. Smokers often use a roach clip to hold it so that the joint can be smoked down to a very small butt. Sometimes marijuana is baked into cookies or brownies. Less THC is absorbed when it is eaten than when it is smoked. To deliver the THC more efficiently to the brain, some people use pipes or special tubes called bongs or rush tubes.

Another way of smoking marijuana involves cigars. Cigars are sliced open and the tobacco is replaced with marijuana. The result is a "blunt." When a "blunt" is smoked while drinking a 40 ounce bottle of malt liquor, the slang term for it is "B-40."

Damaging Results

Recent studies have confirmed that marijuana causes physical and psychological changes in the body. Marijuana contains over 400 different chemicals including tar and carbon monoxide that are found in cigarette smoke. Users inhale the unfiltered marijuana smoke deeply into the lungs causing irritation and damage to the respiratory passages.

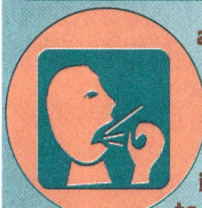

Teens In Control

Marijuana continues to be the most used illegal drug in the United States. However, a little reported fact is that most teens are not and never will be marijuana users. Indeed, fewer than one out of five teenagers say that they use marijuana. Most teens declare their determination to ignore peer pressure and to abstain from experimenting with marijuana or any drugs.

STREET SMART STRATEGIES

KNOWLEDGE POWER: Learn about the dangers of marijuana use.

CORE VALUES: Be a real friend. If your friend has a marijuana problem, encourage him/her to get help.

PROACTION: Take a stand—practice marijuana refusal skills.

BUZZ WORDS

1. Bong — pipe used to produce a stronger effect from marijuana
2. Burn out — term used to describe a person who uses a lot of marijuana and who lacks interest in life
3. Cannabis sativa plant — marijuana plant
4. Hash — strong form of marijuana made from resin of plant
5. Joint — dried leaves, buds, or flowers of the marijuana plant that is rolled and smoked like a cigarette
6. Motivation — determination or will to do something
7. Resin — sticky substance from leaves and flowers of marijuana plant
8. Roach clip — holder for a marijuana cigarette in order to smoke it to a small butt
9. Stoned — high; intoxicated on marijuana
10. THC — tetrahydrocannabinol; mind-altering chemical in marijuana
11. Weed — slang expression for marijuana, joint, pot, chronic, reefer, grass

SHOW IT

PHYSICAL EFFECTS OF MARIJUANA

Marijuana influences the body when it enters the blood stream. The effects are felt within a few minutes and last for a few hours.

BRAIN
Affects short term memory, vision, speech, coordination, decision-making ability

IMMUNE SYSTEM
May interfere with ability to fight disease

HEART
Speeds heart beat up to 50%; danger especially with high blood pressure, heart or circulatory problems

LUNGS
Increased risk of respiratory problems: bronchitis, emphysema, lung cancer

REPRODUCTIVE SYSTEM
Interferes with hormone causing changes in menstrual cycle, sperm production; possible birth defects in newborn

---

Marijuana is used for its mind-altering ability. Short and long term effects are different for each individual. The following changes are not unusual:
- Some users feel happy, relaxed, dreamy, silly or quiet, withdrawn and confused.
- Poor short-term memory
- Delayed reaction time
- Blurred vision and speech
- Poor thinking and decision making abilities
- Driving is particularly dangerous even several hours after the "high" has worn off

WHO IS AT GREATEST RISK?

TEENAGERS
Marijuana changes hormone levels in teens at a time of rapid sexual development. It can cause menstrual irregularities in females, and lowered sperm count in males.

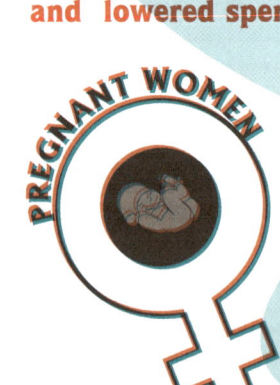

PREGNANT WOMEN
THC passes through placenta to the developing baby causing possibility of birth defects.

NURSING MOTHERS
THC passes from mother's milk to nursing baby.

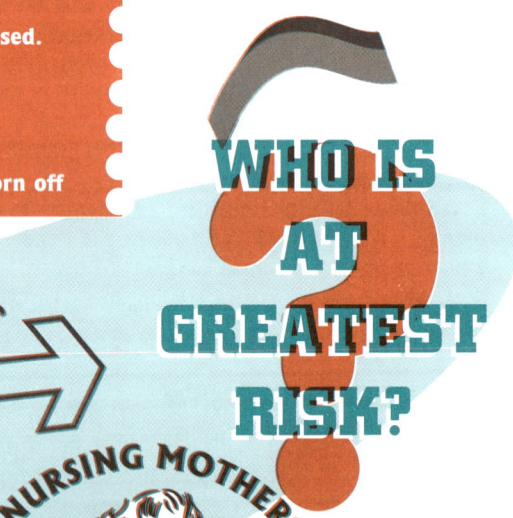

MARIJUANA "BURNOUT"

Marijuana users were the first to use the term "burn out" to describe the characteristics of the heavy marijuana user. A "burn-out" lacks motivation. He or she may be uninterested in their own life or that of others. They may not even answer if someone speaks to them. Most of all, although others clearly see negative changes, they deny they have a problem!

HOOK, LINE, AND SINKER

HOOK: The drugs that get people hooked. **LINE:** The lie that gets them to take the drugs. **SINKER:** The bad results of taking drugs.

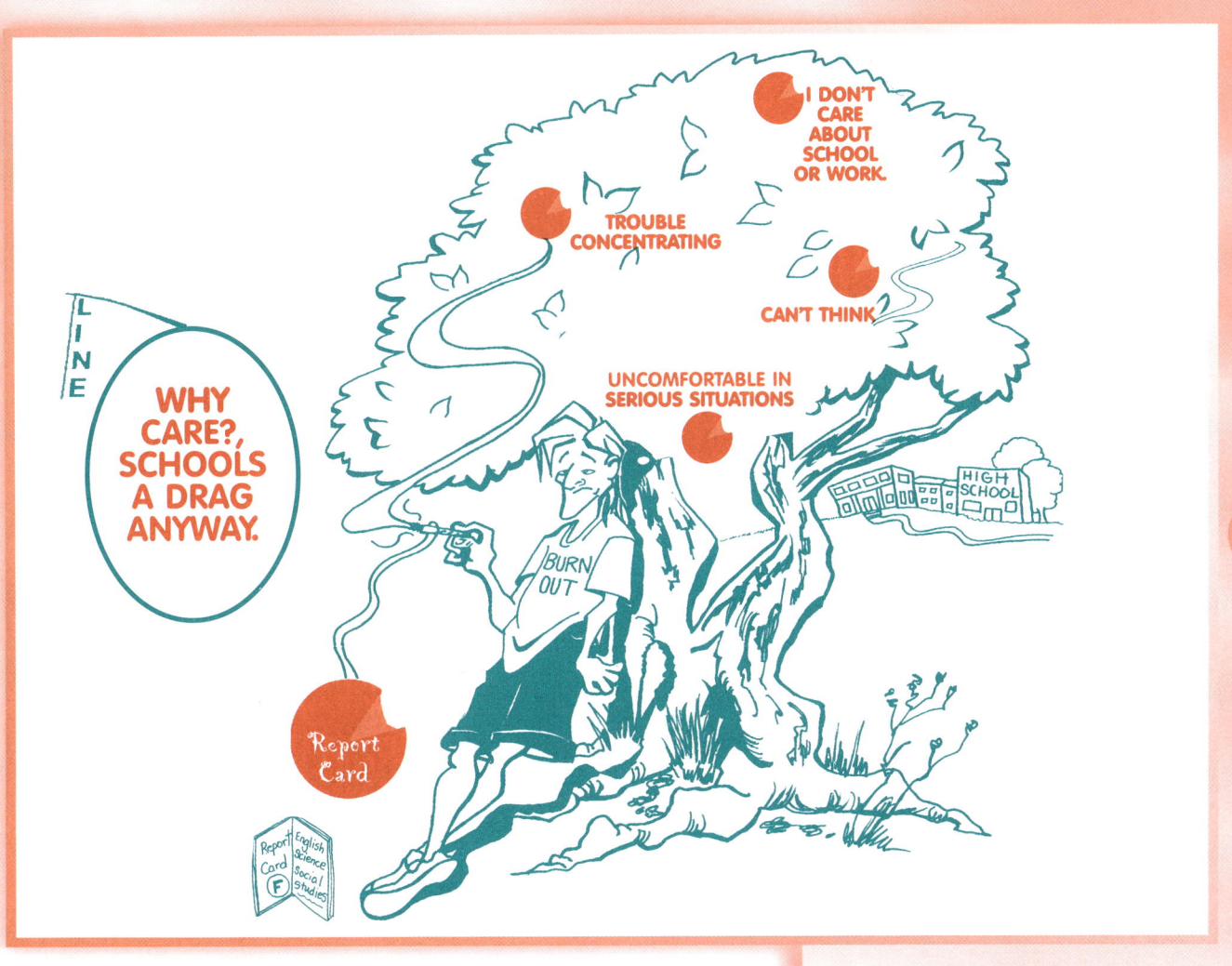

(Cartoon: A "burn out" teen smoking under a tree. Tree labeled with bitten fruits: TROUBLE CONCENTRATING, I DON'T CARE ABOUT SCHOOL OR WORK, CAN'T THINK, UNCOMFORTABLE IN SERIOUS SITUATIONS. LINE flag: WHY CARE?, SCHOOL'S A DRAG ANYWAY. Sinker: Report Card with F.)

THINK ABOUT IT...

Use the cartoon above to answer the following questions:

HOOK — What is the abuser smoking?
_____
_____

LINE — What does the abuser say to convince himself and others not to worry about school?
_____
_____

SINKER — What shows that the abuser has given up on school?
_____
_____

Be Street Smart

Know the law. Marijuana is illegal.

For Advice And Information Call:
National Council on Alcoholism and Drug Dependence (NCADD)

1-800-NCA-Call
or
http://www.ncadd.org

THE PEOPLES PUBLISHING GROUP, 1-800-822-1080. COPYING PROHIBITED BY LAW.

CHECKUP

MATCHING

Column A
1. ___ pot
2. ___ burnout
3. ___ THC
4. ___ experiment
5. ___ motivation

Column B
a. to try something
b. slang for marijuana
c. someone who has smoked pot heavily for a long time
d. tetrahydrocannabinol
e. determination to do something

MULTIPLE CHOICE

1. **How is marijuana used?**
   a. smoked
   b. eaten
   c. both a and b

2. **The mind-altering ingredient in marijuana is**
   a. pot
   b. THC
   c. roach clip

3. **Marijuana is**
   a. legal
   b. illegal
   c. made in a laboratory

4. **A slang term for marijuana is**
   a. weed
   b. bong
   c. roach clip

5. **Marijuana users often**
   a. have poor short-term memory
   b. have better than average memories
   c. have a lot of energy

FILL IN THE BLANKS

joint pipe cannabis clip
eaten smoked THC

Marijuana comes from the _____ plant. The mind-altering ingredient in marijuana is _____. Marijuana is either _____ or _____. Users who smoke marijuana may call the cigarette a _____. They may hold it in a _____ clip so that they can smoke it down to a small butt. They may also smoke it in a _____.

44   MARIJUANA   Street Smarts

TAKE A STAND

Dear Mrs. D.

IMPROVE YOUR REFUSAL SKILLS

Dear Mrs. D.:
Usually parents complain that they think their kids are doing drugs. Not at my house. Both Mom and Dad come home from work and get stoned. Mom "forgets" to make dinner. Dad has me make up stories for his boss about why he can't come to the phone.
The house stinks all the time. Not to mention the mess everywhere because Mom is "too tired" to bother cleaning. I'm embarrassed to have friends visit but I've run out of excuses.

Signed,
Feel like I'm the parent.

Write how you would answer if you were Mrs. D.

Mrs. D. Answers:
_____
_____
_____
_____
_____
_____
_____
_____
_____

Show that you recognize the danger by completing the exercise below.

BJ and Lila were good friends since grade school; they did everything together.
Last month Lila and BJ argued over the boys next door. One of the boys had suggested that Lila and BJ could hang out with him and his brother. Both girls thought the brothers were cute. They were also flattered that the boys liked them and wanted to spend time with them. There was only one problem. Both boys smoked marijuana.
Lila refused to hang out with anyone who did drugs. BJ thought that Lila was silly. They argued. Lila stopped going to BJ's. BJ was lonely and hurt. She began to spend more time with the boys.

1. <u>Underline</u> one sentence that shows how Lila is keeping herself from drug involvement.

2. (Circle) a sentence that shows how BJ could be placing herself at risk.

3. How could Lila maintain a friendship with BJ and still not hang out with druggies? _____
_____

Write the coolest way to say, "No!"

1. **The Offer** "We have time before class, want to share a joint?"

   You say _____
   _____

2. **The Dare** "I bet you don't have the nerve to spike those brownies with 'grass' for the graduation party."

   You say _____
   _____

   BACK OFF

3. **The Threat** "Either you get stoned with us now or you can forget joining us later."

   You say _____
   _____

4. **The Feel Good Approach** "First dates always makes you nervous. Smoke this joint, it will calm you down."

   You say _____
   _____
   _____
   _____

YOUR TURN

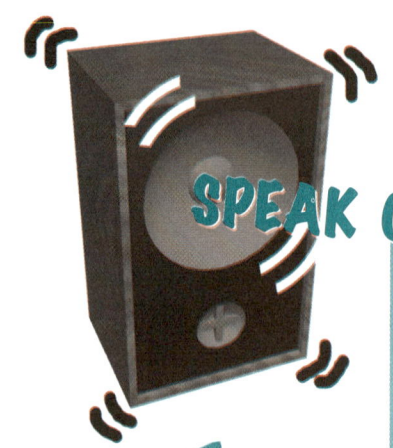

SPEAK OUT

LIGHTS, CAMERA, ACTION!

1. Do you support the idea of "random" or "across the board" drug testing for high school athletes? Why or Why not?

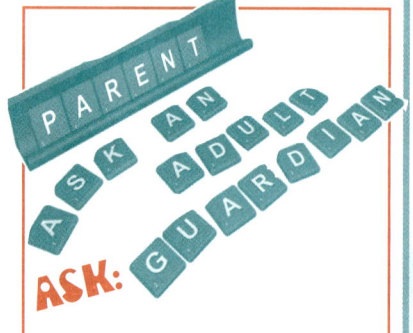

_____
_____

2. If a school district follows a policy of "random" or "across the board" drug testing and finds students that test positive, what should be done? Why?

_____
_____

ASK A PARENT AN ADULT GUARDIAN

Did you have a brother, close relative or friend who smoked weed? Did you tell a grown-up? Why and how?

INTERACT

Setting: The school bus company has a hard time keeping drivers. Your bus driver is new. All the kids know that he smokes cigarettes on the morning runs and weed on the afternoon pick-ups.

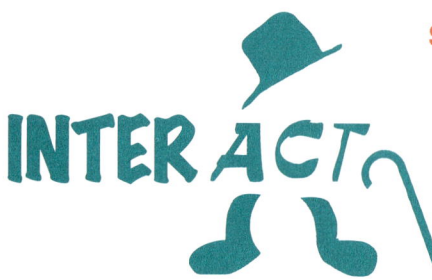

Situation: Most of the kids think he is funny. They know that they can get away with anything when he drives. His driving is pretty wild and so is his behavior.

Solution: You and a few of the "drug-free" kids want to change the situation. Identify the key people that have to be notified. Act out what you would say. Tell how you feel the problem should be solved.

Teen Talk

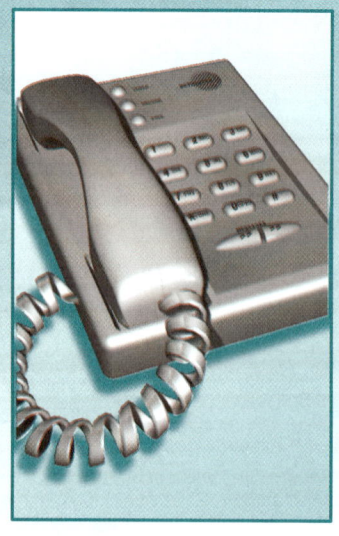

1. What responsibility do teens have if a co-worker at their job is smoking pot on breaks?

_____
_____
_____
_____

2. What would you say/do if your best friend started smoking pot?

_____
_____
_____
_____
_____

STEROIDS

CHAPTER 6

AT THE GYM

"SOMETHING'S HAPPENING TO YOU, MAN. SOMETHING I DON'T LIKE."

It was Thursday night and Manuel was telling his story to the group.

He remembered the first time someone had questioned him about his use of steroids. He had been working out, as usual, when he saw José just standing there, watching him.

"José looked angry. He walked over to me and said, 'Manuel, how much do you weigh now? You look like you've gained forty pounds since Christmas.' Before I could answer, he said, 'You're benching 180! What are you doing to yourself?'"

"What's it to you?" I asked, grabbing him by the chest and yanking him toward me. "You think I want to look like a kid for the rest of my life?"

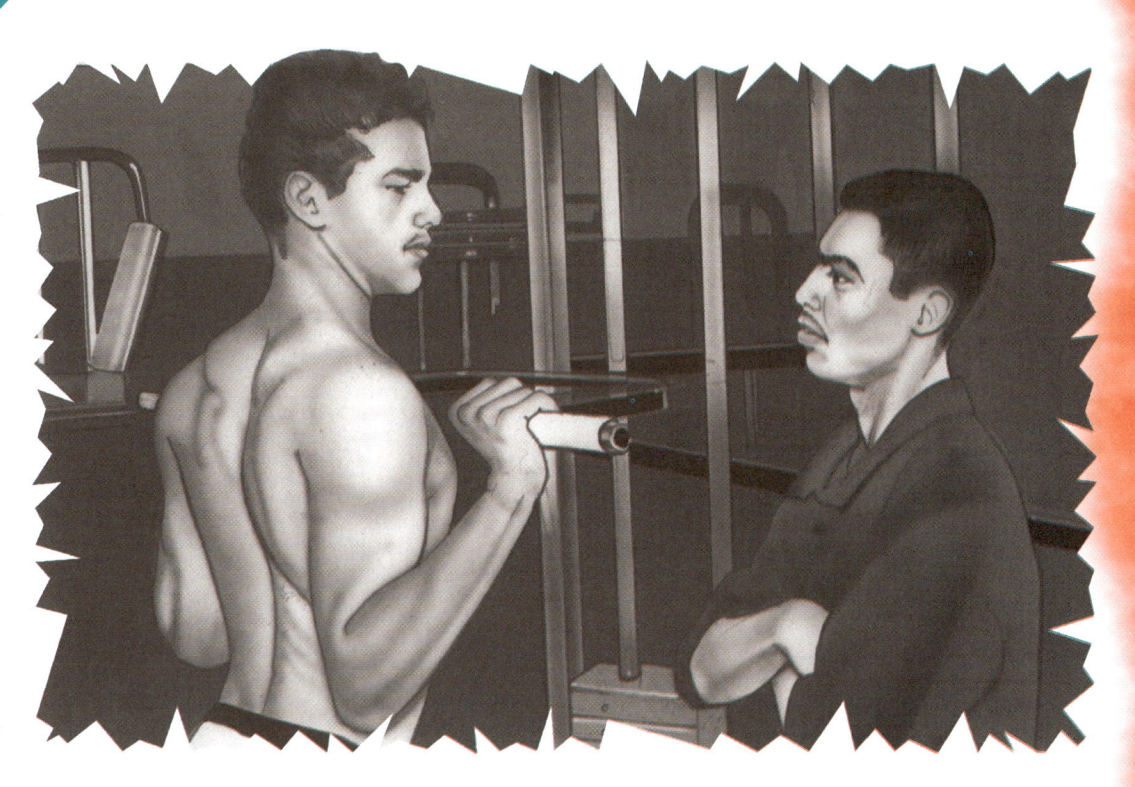

José wouldn't let up. "I thought we were friends, Manuel. Now you act like you're ready to fight me and everyone else. Something's happening to you, man. Something I don't like."

"I finally have girls looking at me. Maybe you're jealous, José."

"Roided Out"

José tried again. "Look, buddy, I'm just trying to tell you the truth. Whatever you're taking is making you look big, but you ain't 'big'. No one wants to be around you. I've heard people bad-mouthing you including some of those girls you're trying to impress."

"I don't believe you. I can

THE PEOPLES PUBLISHING GROUP, 1-800-822-1080. COPYING PROHIBITED BY LAW.

have any one of those girls I want. I see how they look at me."

"Yeah, the girls may be lookin' but you don't hear what they're sayin'. You're 'roided out', Manuel."

On his way out, José added, "One more thing, your breath stinks! Now I've said it, if you don't like it, Manuel, O.K., but I figure friends have got responsibilities to friends."

Manuel looked around the group, then asked, "Can you believe that? He called me a 'roid' and he pretended to be my friend. Who needs friends like that!"

"He must have talked to my girl because she started in on my case. Everyone was sticking their nose into my business. Before you know it, her brother was telling me to take a hike. That did it! I lost it and punched him out good. After what he said, I thought he deserved it."

Manuel looked up. The group wasn't buying it.

Leguero leaned back in his chair and said, "Okay, Manuel, now let's have a little reality check with that story. You have no one to blame but yourself. You broke the law when you attacked your girl's brother and broke up their home. To live in this town, you have to live by its rules. That's why the judge ordered you to pay for the damages."

Real Friends

Manuel's eyes were glued to the floor.

"Manuel, look at me," Mrs. D. ordered. "We've known each other for years. You've called on me as a friend. Well, friends don't always say the things we want to hear. Real friends say what they feel needs to be said. José was a friend to you. He was trying to help you in the best way he could."

> YOU GIVE BUT LITTLE WHEN YOU GIVE OF YOUR POSSESSIONS. IT IS WHEN YOU GIVE OF YOURSELF THAT YOU TRULY GIVE.
>
> *Kahlil Gibran*

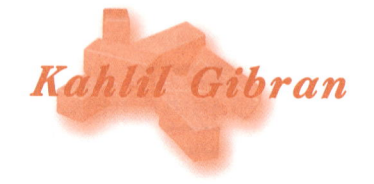

TELL IT

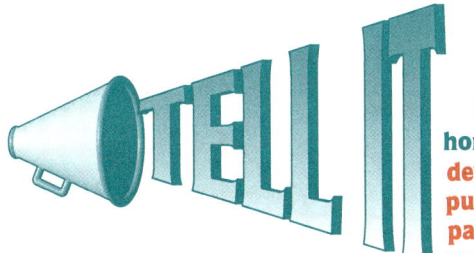

Be Real!

Testosterone is the male hormone that causes boys to develop into men. During puberty, more testosterone passes into the blood stream causing muscles and body hair to develop and the voice to deepen. This is the way a male's body develops naturally. In females, testosterone is also produced naturally, but in smaller amounts.

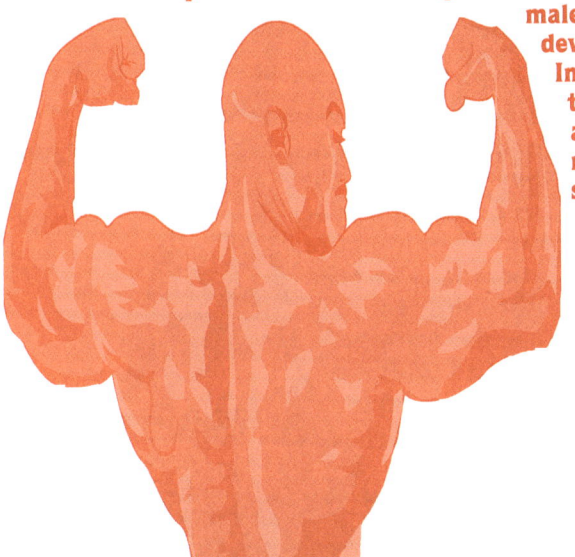

Not For Real!

Anabolic steroids are artificial substances that change the natural way the body grows and develops. These dangerous drugs interfere with normal body development.

Anabolic steroid users take large amounts of these synthetic substances. Some steroids are taken orally as pills or capsules. Some are injected by hypodermic needle deep into the muscles.

Fit?

Steroid users want a quick fix to obtain a developed body. Abusers who work out, may become "ripped." This means that their muscles become clearly defined in a short period of time.

Or Not So Fit?

Steroid abuse has some very dangerous side effects. Abusers may develop bad acne, bad breath, lose hair, and have heart and liver damage. Use of steroids by pre-teens and developing teens may cause bones to stop growing naturally. These teens may have stunted growth. Others have rapid weight gain.

Any steroid abuser who shares needles with other abusers, is at increased risk for AIDS.

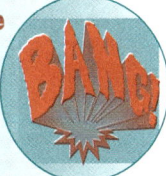

All In The Mind!

Chemicals in steroids cause mood swings and roid rages (sudden aggressive behavior). Abusers may become violent for no apparent reason. They can be dangerous to themselves and to those around them.

STREET SMART STRATEGIES

KNOWLEDGE POWER: Learn about the dangers of steroid abuse.
CORE VALUES: Include exercise in your daily activities. Shortcuts don't work!
PROACTION: Take a stand—practice steroid refusal skills.

BUZZ WORDS

1. Aggressive — hostile, striking out at someone or something
2. AIDS — Acquired Immune Deficiency Syndrome
3. Anabolic steroid — chemical taken internally to promote weight gain and muscle growth
4. Artificial — not natural, man-made
5. Blanks — slang word "false" steroids
6. Dependence — relying or counting on someone or something
7. Hormone — chemical made by the glands of the body
8. Interfere — to prevent or get in the way of
9. Joy rider — person who abuses steroids to looked "ripped"
10. Ripped — increased muscle definition of body builder
11. Roid rages — uncontrolled burst of anger
12. Sterile — unable to produce children
13. Stunted — prevented from growing or developing properly
14. Synthetic — not natural; man-made
15. Testosterone — male hormone

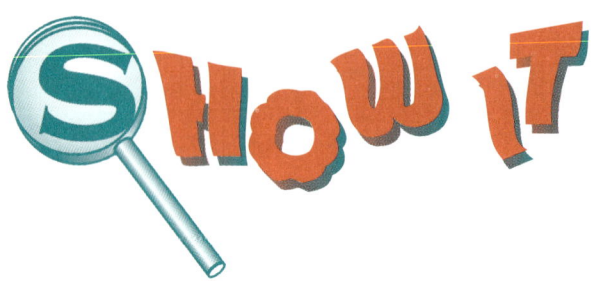

Show it

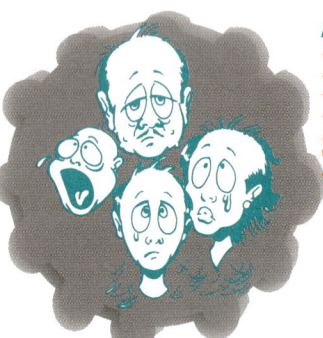

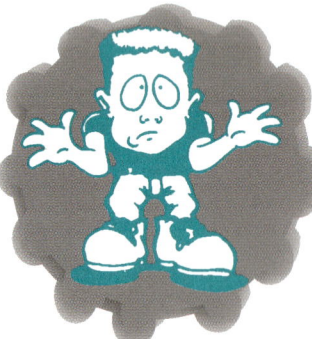

Some people will do almost anything to look good. Teens may become involved with steroids to compete in sports, for the attention of peers, or to improve the way that their body looks. They think that they can get the "perfect body" they imagine. People who take steroids for the muscular "ripped" or "cut" look are called "joy-riders." To make money, some people sell blanks or fake steroids. Blanks are illegal.

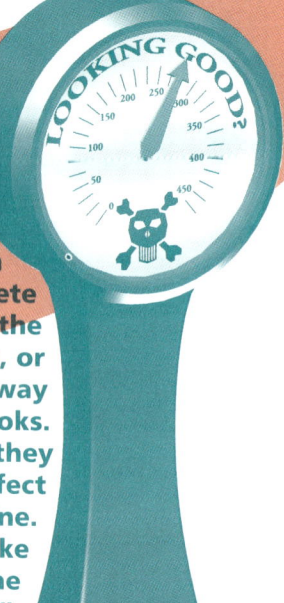

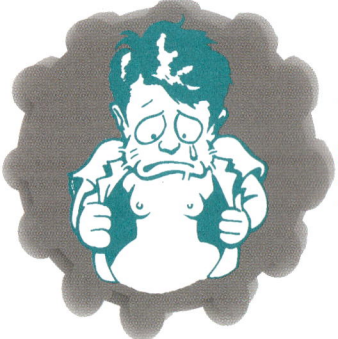

VISIBLE PHYSICAL EFFECTS

ALL USERS
Loss of hair
Early baldness
Severe acne
Yellow eyes and skin

PRE-TEENS
Stunted growth

TEEN/ADULT MALES
Shrinking testicles
Female-type breasts

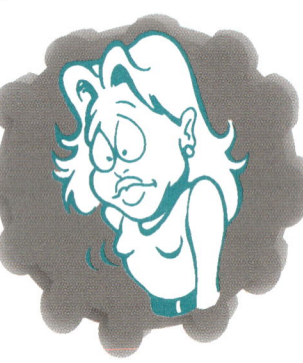

TEEN/ADULT FEMALES
Shrinking breasts
Facial hair growth

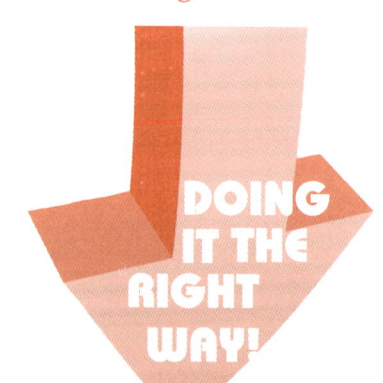

OTHER PHYSICAL EFFECTS

VISIBLE PHYSICAL EFFECTS

Heart damage, heart attacks
Persistent bad breath
High risk of AIDS for those injecting steroids

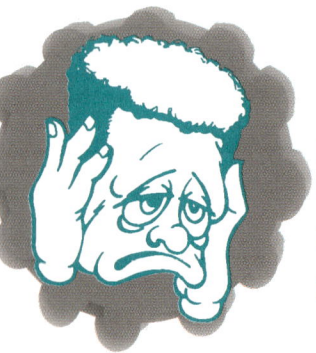

Depression
Violent behavior
Mood swings

DOING IT THE RIGHT WAY!

Athletic excellence has been achieved for centuries without the use of drugs. Today, an increasing number of athletes are enjoying the challenge and reward of developing naturally. They know that good nutrition, exercise, and hard work makes them physically and mentally fit. Cheating by taking drugs may give the appearance of physical fitness, but abusers are risking their health.

HOOK, LINE, AND SINKER

HOOK: The drugs that get people hooked. **LINE:** The lie that gets them to take the drugs. **SINKER:** The bad results of taking drugs.

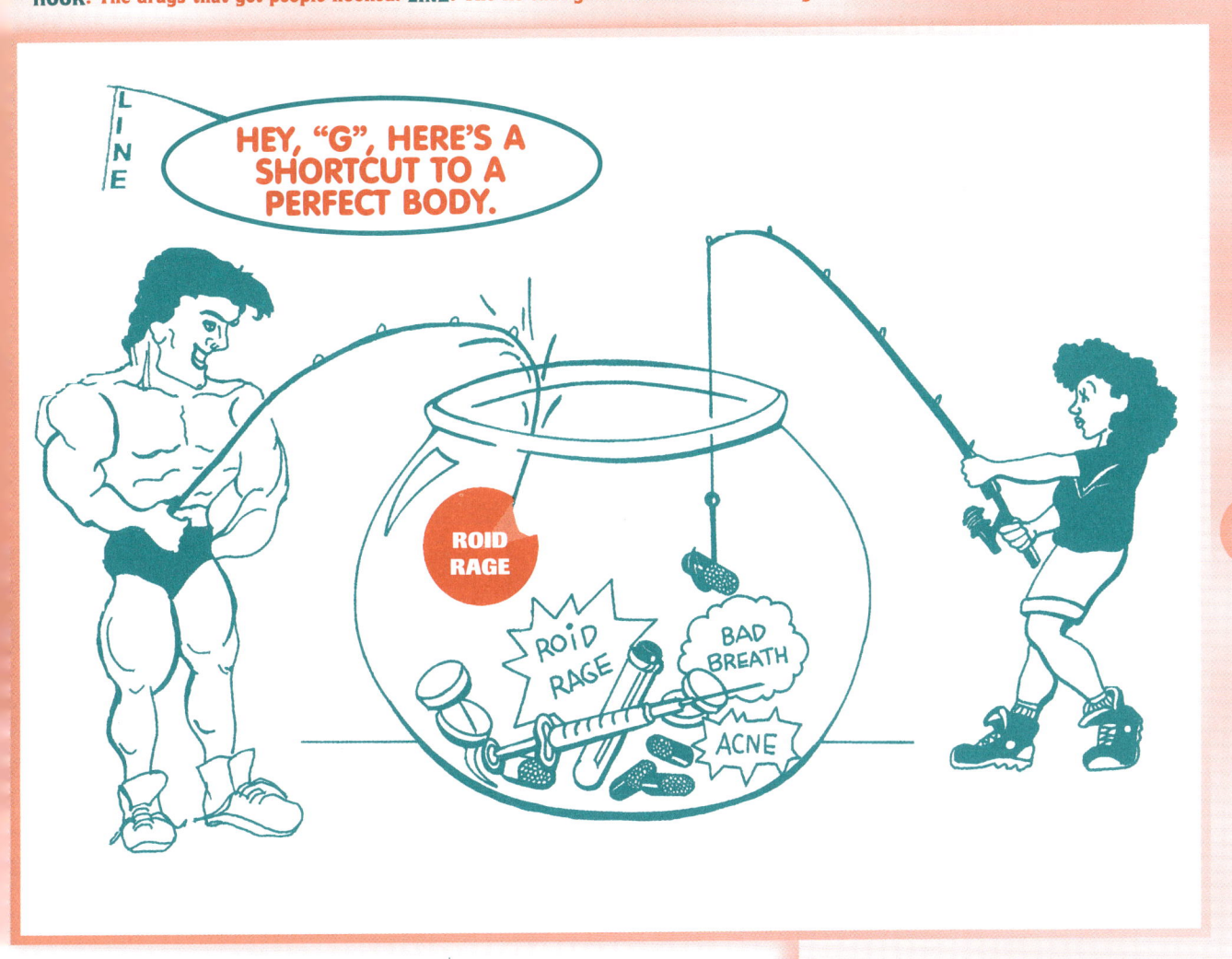

> LINE: "HEY, 'G', HERE'S A SHORTCUT TO A PERFECT BODY."

(ROID RAGE, BAD BREATH, ACNE)

THINK ABOUT IT...

Use the cartoon above to answer the following questions:

HOOK: What drug promises a shortcut to a perfect body?

LINE: What line encourages abuse?

SINKER: What side effect can hurt abusers and those around them?

Be Street Smart

Avoid tempting shortcuts. Exercise is the safe way to build muscle.

For Advice And Information Call:
1-800-622-2255
Action/Pride
Drug Information System

THE PEOPLES PUBLISHING GROUP, 1-800-822-1080. COPYING PROHIBITED BY LAW.

CHECKUP

MATCHING

Column A	Column B
1. ___ "roid rage"	a. side effect of steroid abuse for females
2. ___ larger breasts	b. side effect of steroid abuse for males
3. ___ smaller breasts	c. uncontrolled anger
4. ___ sterile	d. rely on something
5. ___ depend	e. unable to have children

FILL IN THE BLANKS

**angry   heart   shrink   anabolic   yellow
muscles   behavior   dangerous   smaller**

_____ steroids are illegal drugs. People take them to develop their _____. Steroid use is _____. Steroids can damage a person's _____ and/or cause heart attacks. They can damage a person's liver and make skin and eyes turn _____. Sometimes they even make a man's testicles _____.

In a woman, they can cause _____ breasts. They may even make it impossible for a couple to have children. Steroids can also change a person's _____. Some steroid users can get very _____ without good reason.

MULTIPLE CHOICE

1. How are steroids taken?
   a. injection
   b. capsules and tablets
   c. both a and b

2. Anabolic steroids act like:
   a. male hormones
   b. aspirin
   c. vitamin pills

3. Steroids can cause:
   a. muscles to shrink
   b. violent behavior
   c. a stronger heart

4. Some people abuse steroids to:
   a. build muscles
   b. think faster
   c. eat less

5. The best way to build muscles is:
   a. proper diet and exercise
   b. increasing the amount of food eaten
   c. taking steroids

TAKE A STAND

Dear Mrs. D.

IMPROVE YOUR REFUSAL SKILLS

Dear Mrs. D.:
I've been at Jefferson High for almost a year. Every day it's the same thing, I get hassled on the way to school. Once at school, I have to sneak around and try to avoid two bullies who "shake me down" for my lunch money.

Andre is selling "super roids". He swears I won't have to worry about those guys any more if I take them.

I know they're not good for me, but getting beaten up isn't either.

Signed,
Black and blue and unsure what to do

Write how you would answer if you were Mrs. D.

Mrs. D. Answers:
_____
_____
_____
_____
_____
_____
_____
_____

Show that you recognize the danger by completing the exercise below.

Sam listened to his mom and dad discussing his football game over their cocktails. They always talked about how he wasn't as good an athlete as Joey. They didn't think his workouts were enough to get him in shape. They wondered if there was something they could get him that would build him up.

After each game, they got on his case. Couldn't he do better? Didn't he think it was time he started remembering he was Joey's brother? Didn't he think it was time that he started playing like a real athlete?

1. Write a sentence that tells how you think Sam felt.
   _____

2. <u>Underline</u> two sentences that show how Sam's parents put Sam at risk for drug abuse.

3. What might Sam say to stop his parents from this behavior?
   _____

Write the coolest way to say, "No!"

1. **The Offer** "We've got the best team ever. Jerry has some 'roids' for you that will guarantee your success."

   You say _____
   _____

2. **The Dare** "I used steroids and my muscles grew. The girls love my new look. What are you afraid of?"

   You say _____
   _____

   BACK OFF

3. **The Threat** "Sally, you're holding the track team back. If you don't think enough of your team to help them win by taking these steroid capsules, then you can forget hanging out with us!"

   You say _____
   _____

4. **The Feel Good Approach** "The 'roids' will build you up so you'll never look scrawny again."

   You say _____
   _____

YOUR TURN

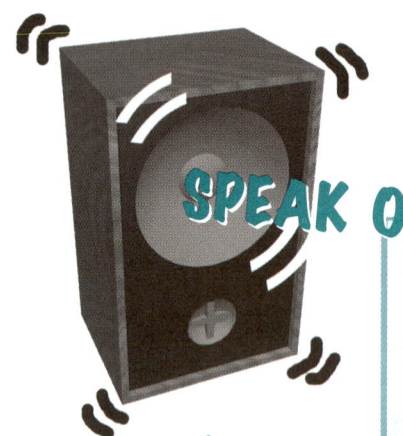

SPEAK OUT

1. Pressure to win by coaches, parents, and friends encourages some teens to take "short cuts" in training. How can coaches increase team performance while discouraging steroid abuse?

_____
_____

2. Strict rules by major sports organizations aim to eliminate steroid abuse by athletes. What punishment would you recommend for athletes who abuse steroids?

_____
_____

PARENT — ASK AN ADULT GUARDIAN

ASK: How much more pressure is put on kids today to excel in athletics than when you were growing up? How did you deal with pressure when you were a teen?

INTERACT

Setting: You are a trained weight-lifter. Because of your training and professional attitude, you have been asked to lead a class in junior high weight-lifting. You know that some of the people in your gym have used steroids.

Situation: After two months of hard work you notice that three weight-lifters (two males and one female) have been building muscle at a much quicker rate than the rest of the class. Although you cannot prove it, you suspect they have been taking steroids.

Solution: After Friday's workout, you excuse the rest of the class and ask these three members to stay back for a "little talk." You are more interested in teaching "responsible safe behavior" than punishment. Act out the scene.

Teen Talk

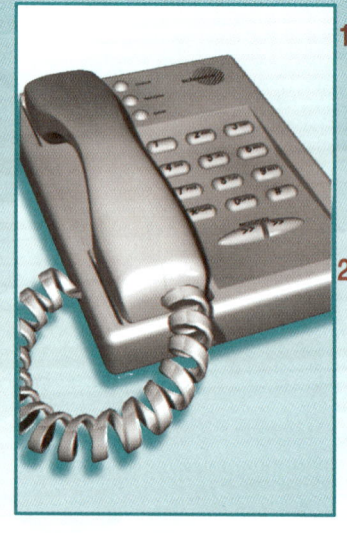

1. Rick, your best friend, hopes to play varsity football but he is worried about making the team. The coach has asked him to do some weight-lifting to build up his muscles. He tells you he is thinking of taking steroids. He asks your advice. What do you tell him?

2. Jo Ann is a member of your gymnastic team. She lifts weights for strength training. Lately you notice changes; she is growing facial hair and the least little thing makes her violent. You suspect she is using steroids. You worry for her, but also for your team. What do you do?

COCAINE

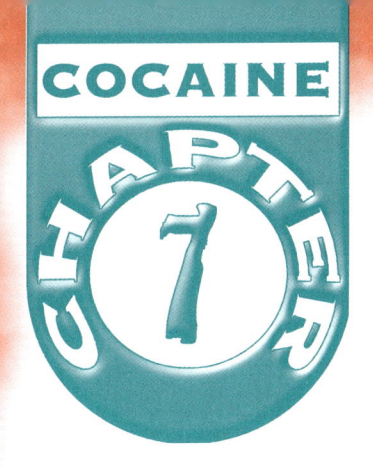

CHAPTER 7

ONE-WAY TICKET TO NOWHERE

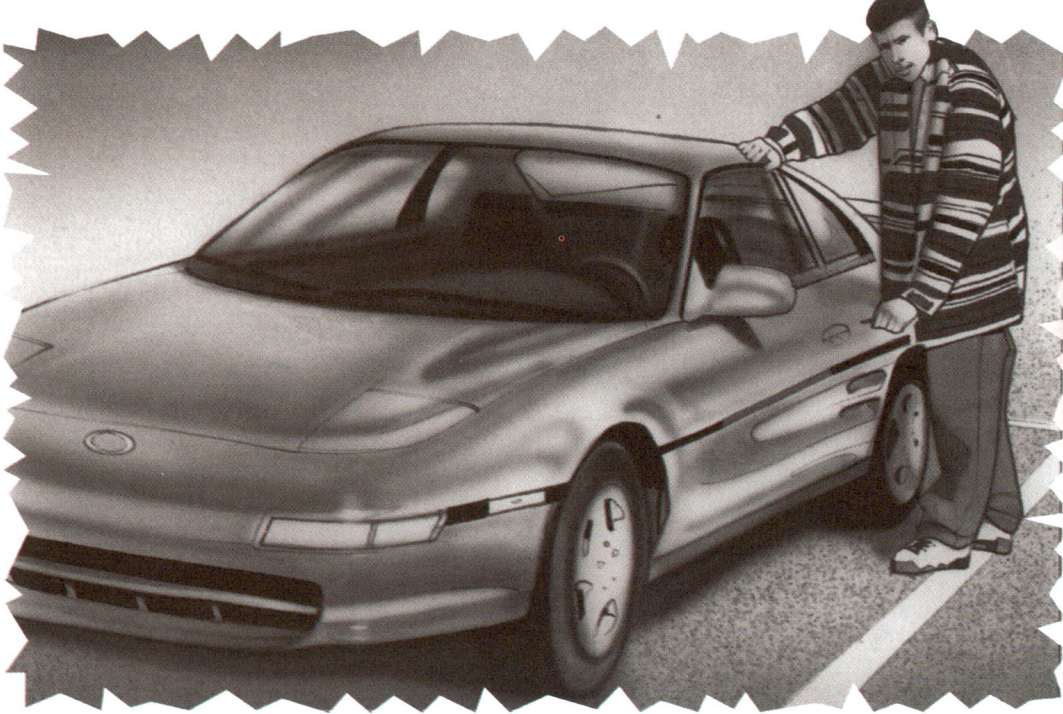

"*This is a free country ... I can come and go as I please*"

"You know, Leguero," Mrs. D. stormed, "that new court placement, John...what's-his-name, really ticks me off.

"He's only been with us for a week and he's always bragging about his money and putting people down. Sometimes I wish the kids would get on his case. I have a hard time with people who think they're better than everyone else!" Mrs. D. asserted.

"He's living proof that money can be a curse," laughed Leguero. He was searching through a mess of papers. "Now where is my note-pad? Hmm, did I leave it home on my dresser," Leguero mumbled, still not paying attention.

Annoyed, Mrs. D. continued, "Leguero, I'm talking about a serious matter here and you won't stop and listen."

Leguero stood up. He put his hands on his hips and looked directly at Mrs. D. "I agree about John. He is a pain. He never shuts up about all his money. Furthermore, I'm not convinced he's clean or has any intention of staying off cocaine."

Mrs. D. agreed. "That's my point. If he's still using cocaine, he can't stay with us."

Attitude Check

"My biggest concern, though, is what he's doing to the "No-Mores"

THE PEOPLES PUBLISHING GROUP, 1-800-822-1080. COPYING PROHIBITED BY LAW.

55

attitude. I think we have to warn him that unless he makes an effort to work with us, he's gone." Leguero looked out the window. "We won't have long to wait. He just pulled up in his fancy car."

John slammed the door behind him and walked toward Leguero and Mrs. D. He reached over and tossed a book down on the table. "See, I told you I could get my own copy. I don't need to share with the group!"

"Hello John," Mrs. D. said pointedly. "We were just talking about you. Sit down. We have some things to straighten out."

"Forget it, I've got a date. I'll see you later."

Strike Out

John almost made it to the door when Leguero stepped in front of him. "You must not have heard the lady. She said "sit down!"

"And just who do you think you are?" flared John. "Nobody, not even my dad, talks to me that way. This is a free country and I can come and go as I please."

John grabbed his book from the table and rushed through the door. Before Leguero could respond, John jumped into his car, floored the gas pedal and sped down the street.

Leguero turned to Mrs. D., "John just wrote his one way ticket back to the judge. He doesn't want our help."

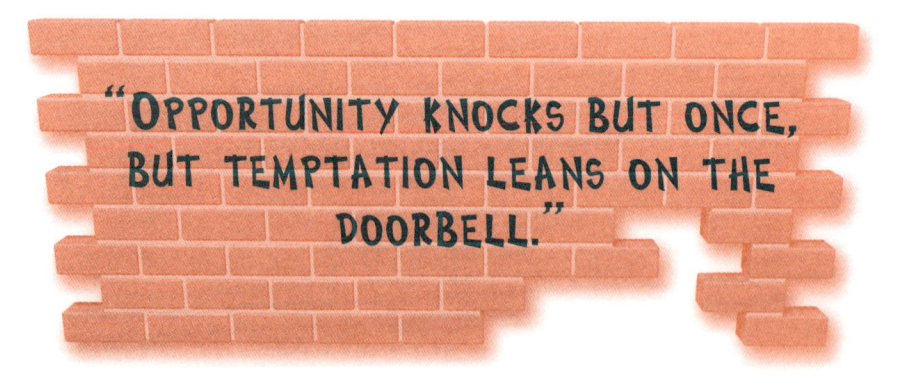

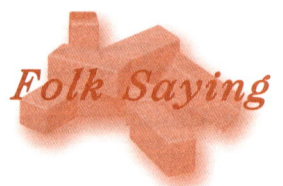

"OPPORTUNITY KNOCKS BUT ONCE, BUT TEMPTATION LEANS ON THE DOORBELL."

Folk Saying

TELL IT

Countries Ban Use

Cocaine comes from the Central and South American coca plant. Before people realized how addictive cocaine was, it was used in cough medicines and even some cola soft drinks! Now it is known to be physically and psychologically addictive and very dangerous. Modern processing techniques have made it so powerful that countries throughout the world have banned its use.

The leaves of the plant are processed to make a strong white powder, often called "snow." This fine powder, or "coke," controls mind and body. Cocaine addiction is so overwhelming that abusers will do anything and pay any price to feed their habit.

Dealers know their customers will buy whatever they sell them. They often "cut" the cocaine by adding cheaper ingredients to the cocaine powder to stretch it so they'll have more cocaine to sell. Abusers risk their lives as well as arrest to sell or buy cocaine. There is no way to know what the dealers have used to cut the cocaine or how strong it is.

Cocaine abusers have sometimes been called status conscious. They have been known to exhibit pride in being able to afford cocaine addiction. At one time it was fashionable to show off your addiction by snorting cocaine through tightly rolled 100 dollar bills!

A Double-Crosser

Users inhale or snort cocaine through the nose, or inject it into a vein. Sometimes it is smoked in a form called freebase or mixed with tobacco or marijuana and smoked.

Cocaine in any form speeds up the nervous system. The heart beats faster, blood pressure increases, and blood vessels get narrower. This combination causes a high or rush—an intense feeling of pleasure.

It also creates stress on blood vessels. Sometimes it causes a weakness or break in the blood vessel wall. If this occurs in or near the heart, a heart attack is likely. When it happens in the brain it can cause a stroke that often leaves the person paralyzed.

Whether cocaine is snorted, injected or smoked, it stimulates the central nervous system to produce a powerful rush. This rush can also result in anxiety and paranoia. Some abusers try to offset the nervous power of the cocaine stimulation by using alcohol as a depressant. The abuser takes a depressant such as wine or beer to calm down from the cocaine anxiety. The combination of the "up" from cocaine and the "down" from a depressant leads to double trouble. The abuser's body suffers from the effects from both drugs. Frequently, the abuser becomes addicted to both drugs.

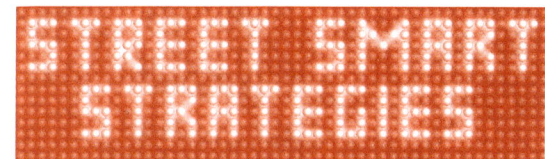

STREET SMART STRATEGIES

KNOWLEDGE POWER: Learn about the dangers of cocaine abuse.
CORE VALUES: Get involved with life, learn new skills. Associate with positive people.
PROACTION: Take a stand—practice cocaine refusal skills.

BUZZ WORDS

1. Anxiety — a feeling of tension, stress, or worry
2. Cocaine — illegal drug made from coca leaves; powder called "coke" or "snow"
3. Convulsions — uncontrollable body movements
4. Crash — the low feeling or depression present when the drug wears off
5. Dealer — person who sells drugs
6. Freebase — smokable form of cocaine
7. Rush — an intense feeling of pleasure
8. Snort — to inhale through the nose
9. Stimulant — a drug that speeds up body activities such as heartbeat
10. Stroke — condition in which brain and nerve tissue die due to poor blood supply. This may cause loss of speech or paralysis
11. Tolerance — ability to withstand more of a drug without feeling the effects

SHOW IT

THE HIGH AND LOW OF COCAINE

HIGH — Feeling of Energy

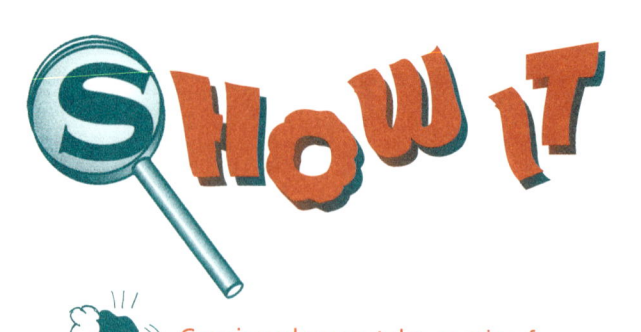

Cocaine abusers take cocaine for the tremendous "high" and feeling of power it causes. That feeling lasts about five to thirty minutes.

CRASH — Feeling of Depression

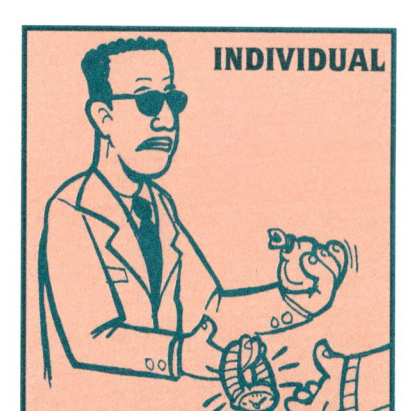

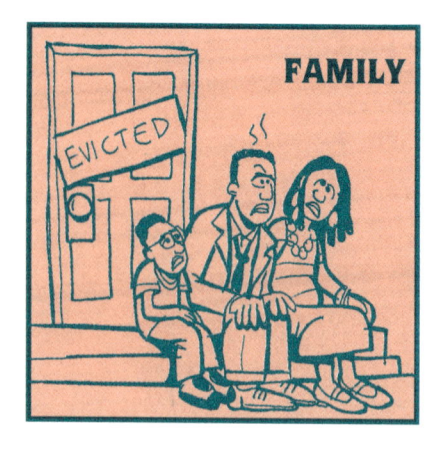

Afterward, many people crash. They suffer severe depression and anxiety and return to cocaine to feel high again. A tolerance develops in the abuser's body causing the need for larger and larger amounts of cocaine in order to get high.

CRAVING — Demands More Cocaine

Many abusers damage the lining in the nose. Frequent cocaine use often results in convulsions, hallucinations and other serious mental problems. Cocaine can cause death when it interferes with the brain's control over heart and lung functions. Cocaine abusers often make poor decisions involving sex. Their action increases the spread of AIDS and other sexually transmitted diseases.

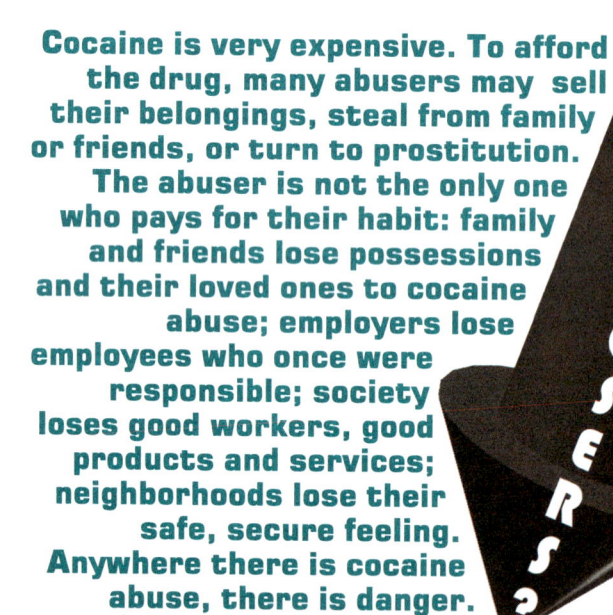

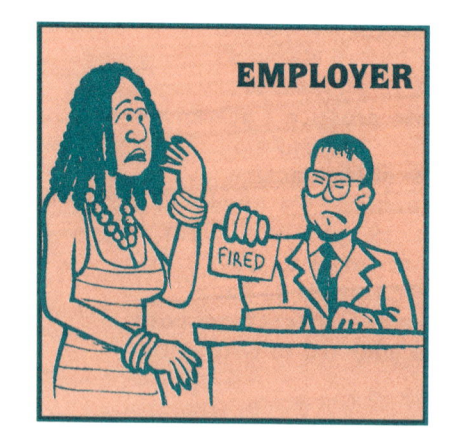

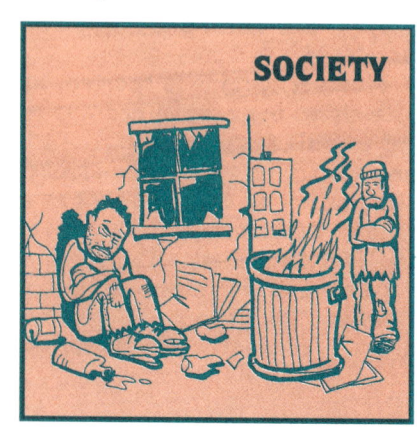

WHO ARE THE LOSERS?

Cocaine is very expensive. To afford the drug, many abusers may sell their belongings, steal from family or friends, or turn to prostitution. The abuser is not the only one who pays for their habit: family and friends lose possessions and their loved ones to cocaine abuse; employers lose employees who once were responsible; society loses good workers, good products and services; neighborhoods lose their safe, secure feeling. Anywhere there is cocaine abuse, there is danger.

INDIVIDUAL

FAMILY

EMPLOYER

SOCIETY

COCAINE — Street Smarts

HOOK, LINE, AND SINKER

HOOK: The drugs that get people hooked. **LINE:** The lie that gets them to take the drugs. **SINKER:** The bad results of taking drugs.

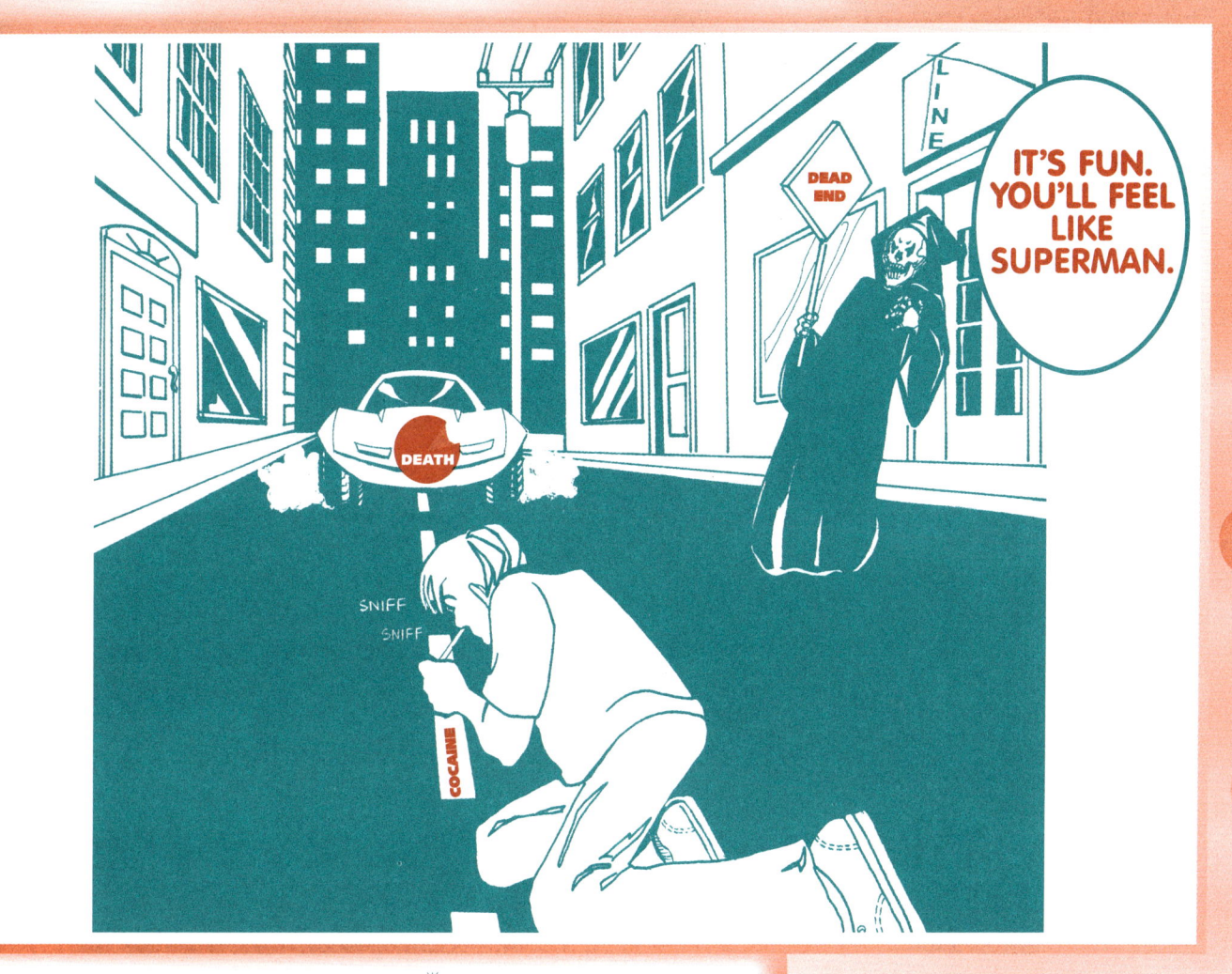

[Cartoon: A person kneels on a city street sniffing cocaine. A car marked "DEATH" approaches, signs read "DEAD END" and "LINE". A grim reaper says "IT'S FUN. YOU'LL FEEL LIKE SUPERMAN."]

THINK ABOUT IT...

Use the cartoon above to answer the following questions:

HOOK
What drug is being snorted?
_____
_____

LINE
What line promotes cocaine abuse?
_____
_____

SINKER
What sinker will overcome the abuser?
_____
_____

Be Street Smart

Addiction and death could occur on even the first use of cocaine.

Don't gamble with your life!

For Advice And Information Call:

1-800-COCAINE

THE PEOPLES PUBLISHING GROUP, 1-800-822-1080. COPYING PROHIBITED BY LAW.

CHECKUP

MATCHING

Column A

1. ___ snow
2. ___ stimulant
3. ___ anxiety
4. ___ stroke
5. ___ "rush"

Column B

a. worried, a feeling of stress
b. may cause paralysis
c. "high" of cocaine
d. slang for cocaine
e. drug that speeds up body functions

FILL IN THE BLANKS

crash   stimulant   inhaled   smoked
injected   rush   snow

Cocaine is a powerful _____. It is sometimes called _____. It is taken in one of three ways: _____, _____, or _____.

A cocaine high is called a _____. The "low" which follows is called a _____.

MULTIPLE CHOICE

1. "Snorting" means
   a. inhaling
   b. exhaling
   c. digesting

2. How long does a cocaine "high" usually last?
   a. about 5-30 minutes
   b. about 3-4 hours
   c. about 3-4 days

3. The cocaine "low" is called:
   a. high
   b. crash
   c. craving

4. Weakened blood vessels caused by cocaine abuse may lead to:
   a. heart attack or stroke
   b. AIDS
   c. cancer

5. Stimulants cause body functions
   a. to slow down
   b. to stay the same
   c. to speed up

TAKE A STAND

Dear Mrs. D.

IMPROVE YOUR REFUSAL SKILLS

Dear Mrs. D.:

I started experimenting with drugs in junior high. A couple of friends would come over on Fridays to "party." Usually we smoked weed or drank beer. A few weeks ago, we tried cocaine.

Now I'm afraid I'm hooked. I want to quit, but cocaine keeps calling me back.

I don't want my parents to find out, but I can't seem to stop wanting and using it. And I don't have enough money to keep buying it. I feel trapped.

Signed,
A "coke-aholic"

Write how you would answer if you were Mrs. D.

Mrs. D. Answers:
_____
_____
_____
_____
_____
_____
_____
_____
_____

Show that you recognize the danger by completing the exercise below.

Joan's friends think her parents are the greatest. Sometimes they chaperone Joan's parties, sometimes they don't. They never say anything when kids "wander" out to their cars for beer. They seem not to notice the smell of weed. In fact, some kids want to have parties at Joan's home because they know that her parents will overlook their drugs use.

Joan thought everything was great until she walked in on her mother doing some coke." Her mother just laughed it off, but Joan feels uneasy.

1. **Underline** a sentence that shows how Joan's parents are encouraging drug abuse.

2. **Circle** one sentence that shows Joan is at risk.

3. What could Joan say to her mother to show her concern? _____
_____
_____

Write the coolest way to say, "No!"

1. **The Offer** These cool guys from the city invite you and your friends over for some 'white heaven.'
   You say _____
   _____

2. **The Dare** "Come on, Al, are you scared to ride the fast lane? Try some coke."
   You say _____
   _____
   _____

   BACK OFF

3. **The Threat** "If partying with 'snow' is too much for you, kid, call a cab and leave."
   You say _____
   _____
   _____

4. **The Feel Good Approach** "Anything that feels this good can't hurt you."
   You say _____
   _____

SPEAK OUT

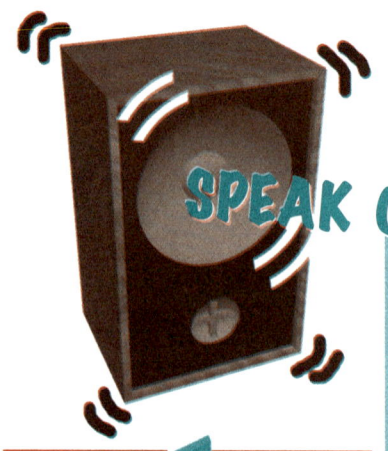

YOUR TURN
LIGHTS, CAMERA, ACTION!

1. Many companies warn job applicants that they will need to pass a drug test before being hired. In what way is this a good idea? Bad idea?

_____
_____

2. What penalty should be given to professional athletes that abuse cocaine?

_____
_____

PARENT ASK AN ADULT GUARDIAN

ASK: Have you ever been around cocaine abuse? How did you handle the situation?

INTERACT

Setting: You're new at school. You're invited to a party by one of the most popular kids: you're "psyched." This is your chance to finally meet some friends.

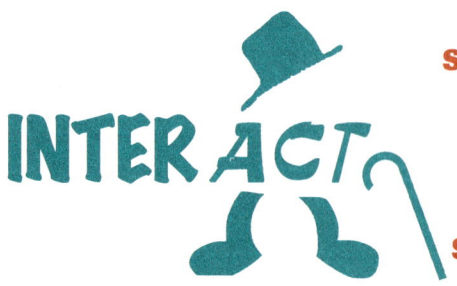

Situation: Amy, the girl you would like to date, invites you into a back room where kids are snorting cocaine through straws. You try to leave, but the "girl of your dreams" puts her arm around you and whispers, "Come on, don't be a drag."

Solution: Act out the scene.

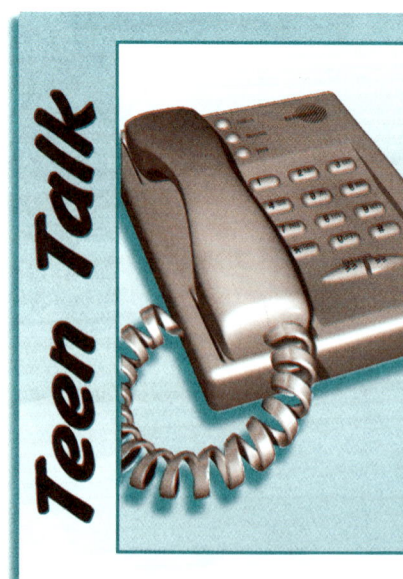

Teen Talk

1. One of the popular guys at school asks you to drop a small package off at George's place. As you take the package, he says, "It's worth $20 to you." Write your first thoughts.

2. What will you do with the package?

_____
_____
_____
_____
_____

62   COCAINE   Street Smarts

CHAPTER 8 — CRACK

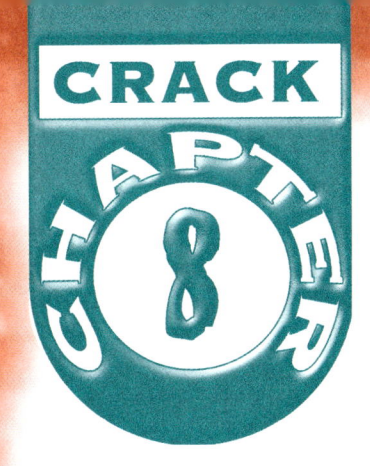

IDENTICAL BUT NOT ALIKE

Pam decided that she was not going to put it off any longer. She put her jacket on and headed to Mr. Rodriguez's grocery store. Maybe Mrs. D. would be there. On previous shopping trips, Pam had noticed the backroom where the "No-Mores" met. Pam knew that Mrs. D. often spent time there with kids. She hoped that Mrs. D. would be there today to talk to her.

If Mrs. D. was surprised, she didn't show it. Her only emotion was a look of delight. She hadn't seen Pam for some time now, even though they were neighbors. Mrs. D. smiled, Outside of the family, I'm probably one of the few people who can tell Pam and her identical twin, Lisa, apart, she thought. Pam's inquiring look made Mrs. D. realize that Pam wanted to talk.

"Tell me, Pam. What is going on?" Mrs. D. asked.

The Sneak

"Oh, Mrs. D., things are really bad. I just don't know what to do about Lisa. Yesterday afternoon I was fixing my hair in the bathroom. It's right next to the bedroom that Lisa and I share. I thought I was alone. Then, I heard a noise in our bedroom. I looked in and saw Lisa at my dresser, with the drawer open."

Mrs. D. listened patiently. She could tell Pam was sorting the events out as she talked.

"Lisa had her headset on so she didn't hear me come up behind her. She

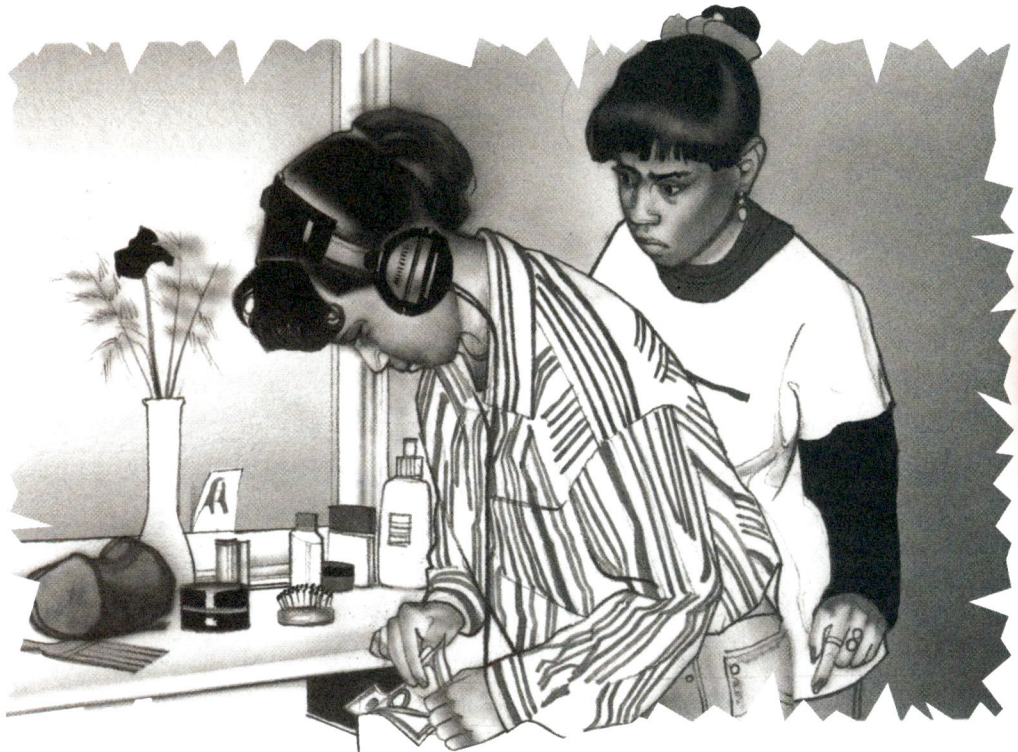

"IT'S MY MONEY, AND YOU'RE STEALING IT!"

was taking the $40 Grandma had given me for my birthday from my drawer! She had folded the bills and was about to stuff them into her pocket. When Lisa realized that I was behind her, she turned and screamed at me, 'Get away from me, you sneak!'"

Pam shook her head in disbelief and continued. "Lisa acted as if I had done something wrong. I couldn't believe it. There she was with my money, and she was blaming me! 'Put my money back,' I yelled. 'What do you think you're doing?'"

Then she said, 'I wasn't taking your money. Why do you always follow me around? Leave me alone!' She put my money into her jeans pocket and ran out of the room."

"It felt like we were strangers," Pam continued. "It's been months since we've done anything together. But if being sisters again means hanging out with a bunch of crackheads, I'd rather be alone."

"Does Lisa think she's addicted to crack?" Mrs. D. asked gently.

"She acts like I'm crazy to think she is addicted to crack. I told her to get real. 'Who does she think she's fooling?' I hear her sneaking out at night. She doesn't take care of herself anymore. And all she thinks about is crack. It's taken over her life."

No More Lies

"I was trying to think what to do when Mr. Green from the supermarket called. Lisa hadn't shown up for work again.

"I thought about going in and covering for her on the job. But I've had enough of the lies. I'm tired of covering up her mistakes. I told Mr. Green Lisa wasn't home. Then I decided to come here to see you."

Mrs. D. reached over and hugged Pam. She was glad that at least this twin was asking for help.

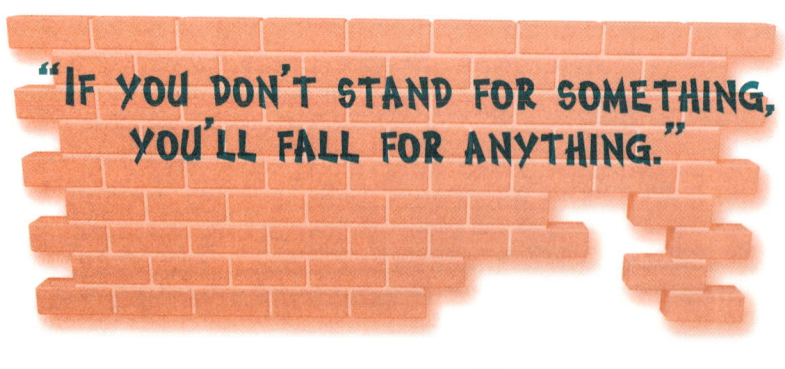

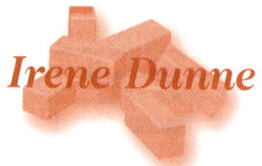

"IF YOU DON'T STAND FOR SOMETHING, YOU'LL FALL FOR ANYTHING."

Irene Dunne

TELL IT

Deadly Twist On an Old Drug

In the 1980s, a new drug began appearing on the streets of major cities. Frequent reports told of crack houses where people bought and smoked the drug. Almost overnight, crack seemed to take over. It destroyed lives and neighborhoods.

Crack is a man-made form of cocaine. Crack is about six times more powerful than cocaine powder. It got its name from the "crackling" sound it makes as it is smoked. Some users call it rock because it looks like small broken pieces of rock. Many crack abusers smoke crack using a glass pipe. A mesh "screen" is pushed down into the pipe. The crack "rocks" are added. The pipe is then heated with a cigarette lighter and the abuser inhales the smoke.

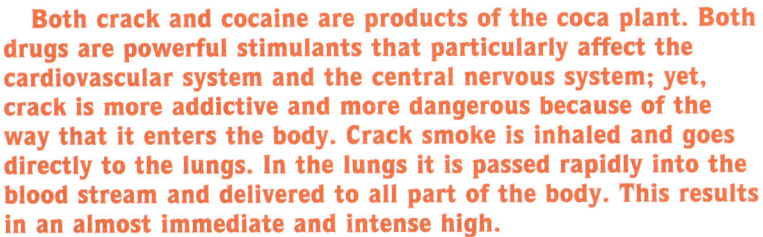

Both crack and cocaine are products of the coca plant. Both drugs are powerful stimulants that particularly affect the cardiovascular system and the central nervous system; yet, crack is more addictive and more dangerous because of the way that it enters the body. Crack smoke is inhaled and goes directly to the lungs. In the lungs it is passed rapidly into the blood stream and delivered to all part of the body. This results in an almost immediate and intense high.

Many crack addicts warn: "Don't ever try crack. Once you start, you'll never stop." Both the abuser and society pay a hish price for the crack addict's addiction. The abuser exchanges his/her life for the crack habit. Society pays the price in violent crime, fatalities from overdose, abandoned or addicted crack babies, skyrocketing health costs, AIDS and STD's. Sadly, society also loses the talents and contributions that the abuser could have made to improve families and communities.

Drug Dealers Delight

Drug dealers love crack. They can sell it in small units, vials, for as little as $5 a hit so that people think it is cheap. More importantly, it is so addictive that new addicts can be made in a few days.

Users report that within seconds they feel an intense high. Less talked about is the equally powerful crash that follows in about fifteen minutes. The intensity of pleasure quickly turns into intense depression, anger, and anxiety.

The memory of the high, especially during the crash, quickly leads to addiction. Because addicted users need a hit so often, crack quickly becomes an expensive habit. Addicts often turn to stealing, dealing, or prostitution to provide the money for its purchase.

Crack causes a high level of dependence. This often leads to "binges." During a binge, abusers smoke crack continuously, trying to eliminate the crash. A binge ends when an addict runs out of money or crack or when he or she passes out.

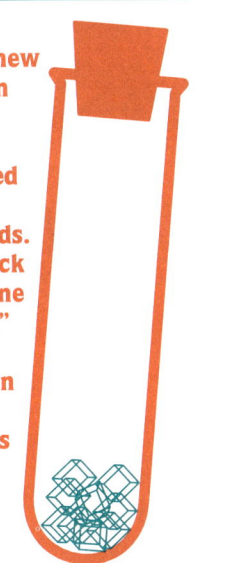

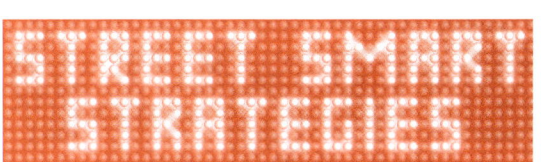

STREET SMART STRATEGIES

KNOWLEDGE POWER: Learn the dangers of crack abuse

CORE VALUES: Don't make excuses for yourself or others. Be responsible for your actions.

PROACTION: Take a stand—practice crack refusal skills.

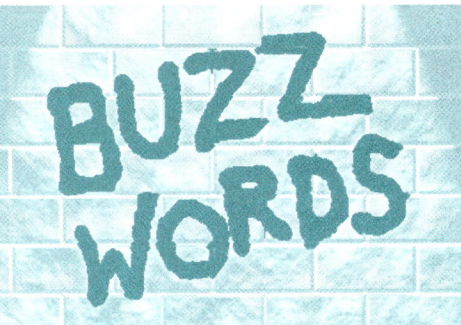

BUZZ WORDS

1. **Binge** — to smoke crack continually until money for crack is gone
2. **Crack** — a "rock" form of cocaine that can be smoked
3. **Crack house** — place where users go to buy and smoke crack
4. **Deformities** — parts of a body not formed properly
5. **Depression** — continued feeling of intense sadness
6. **Hit** — amount of drug taken
7. **Hyperactive** — very active
8. **Insomnia** — sleeplessness
9. **Prostitution** — sale of body in exchange for something (money, sex or drugs)
10. **Rock** — another name for crack
11. **Vial** — plastic container in which crack is sold

Show It

How CRACK Works

When crack is smoked, it is taken directly into the lungs. Tiny air sacs in the lungs pass it into the blood. Within about seven seconds, it reaches the brain and can injure or kill.

Physical Effects

- increased heart beat, blood pressure, even heart attack
- problems breathing, sore throat, scratchy voice
- severe headaches, vomiting
- tremors (shakes), seizures, stroke
- insomnia
- no energy
- dependence on crack
- weight loss due to lack of interest in food

Psychological Effects

- tremendous high followed quickly by "crash" (strong depression, fear, feeling of worthlessness)
- quick anger that may lead to violent behavior
- fear that something bad will happen; guilt for being addicted, treating others badly and stealing
- reduced concentration, poor thinking
- dependence on crack
- mental illness
- loss of interest in friends and activities
- rapid mood changes

Show It: The Facts

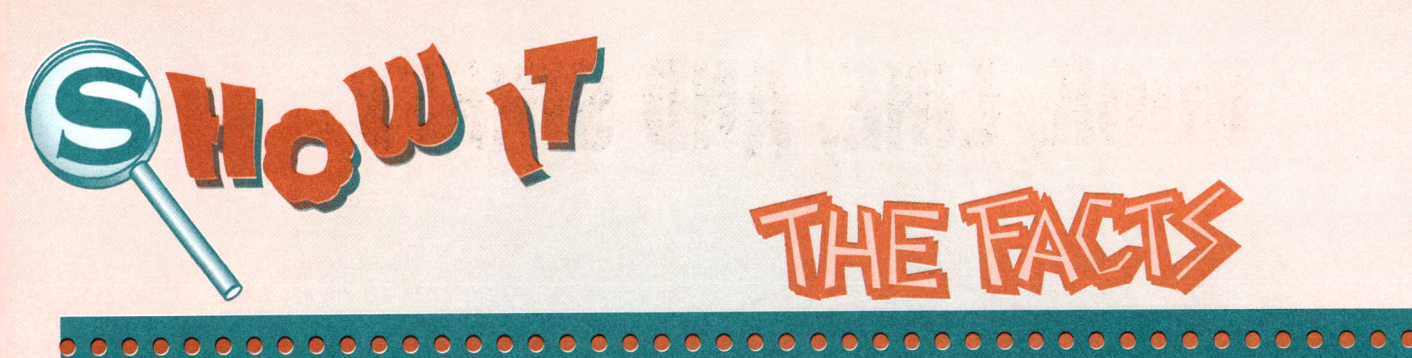

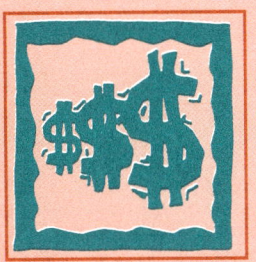

COSTS
Crack starts cheap but ends up costing a lot because the user needs more of the drug to get and stay high.

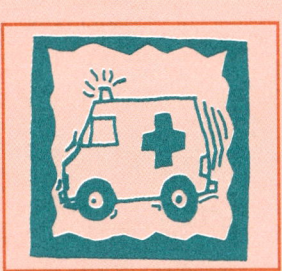

FATALITIES
Crack can cause a heart attack or cause a person to stop breathing. This can happen even the first time it is used.

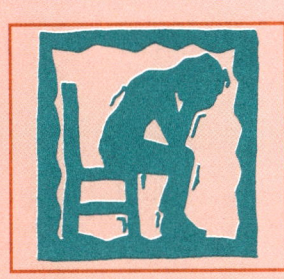

ADDICTS
Crack is considered one of the most addicting drugs in the United States today.

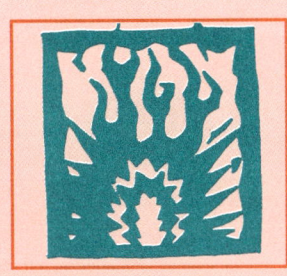

EXPLOSIONS
Changing cocaine into crack involves using dangerous chemicals. These added substances can catch fire or explode.

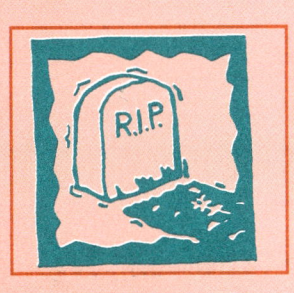

CRIMES
Many people are murdered each year in robberies for crack money. Most are innocent victims.

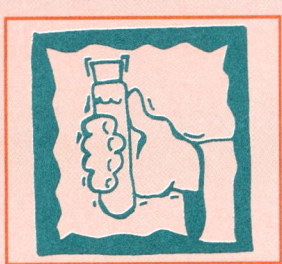

TESTS
Many employers test for drugs. Some tests can detect crack even a month after it was used.

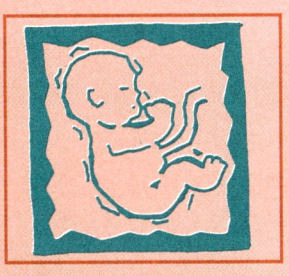

VICTIMS
Unborn babies are often victims of their mother's addiction. Taken during pregnancy, crack can cause birth defects or deformities. Doctors report that "crack babies" are often extremely hyperactive, fearful and difficult to care for. As "crack babies" grow older, they may have learning and behavior difficulties.

HOOK, LINE, AND SINKER

HOOK: The drugs that get people hooked. **LINE:** The lie that gets them to take the drugs. **SINKER:** The bad results of taking drugs.

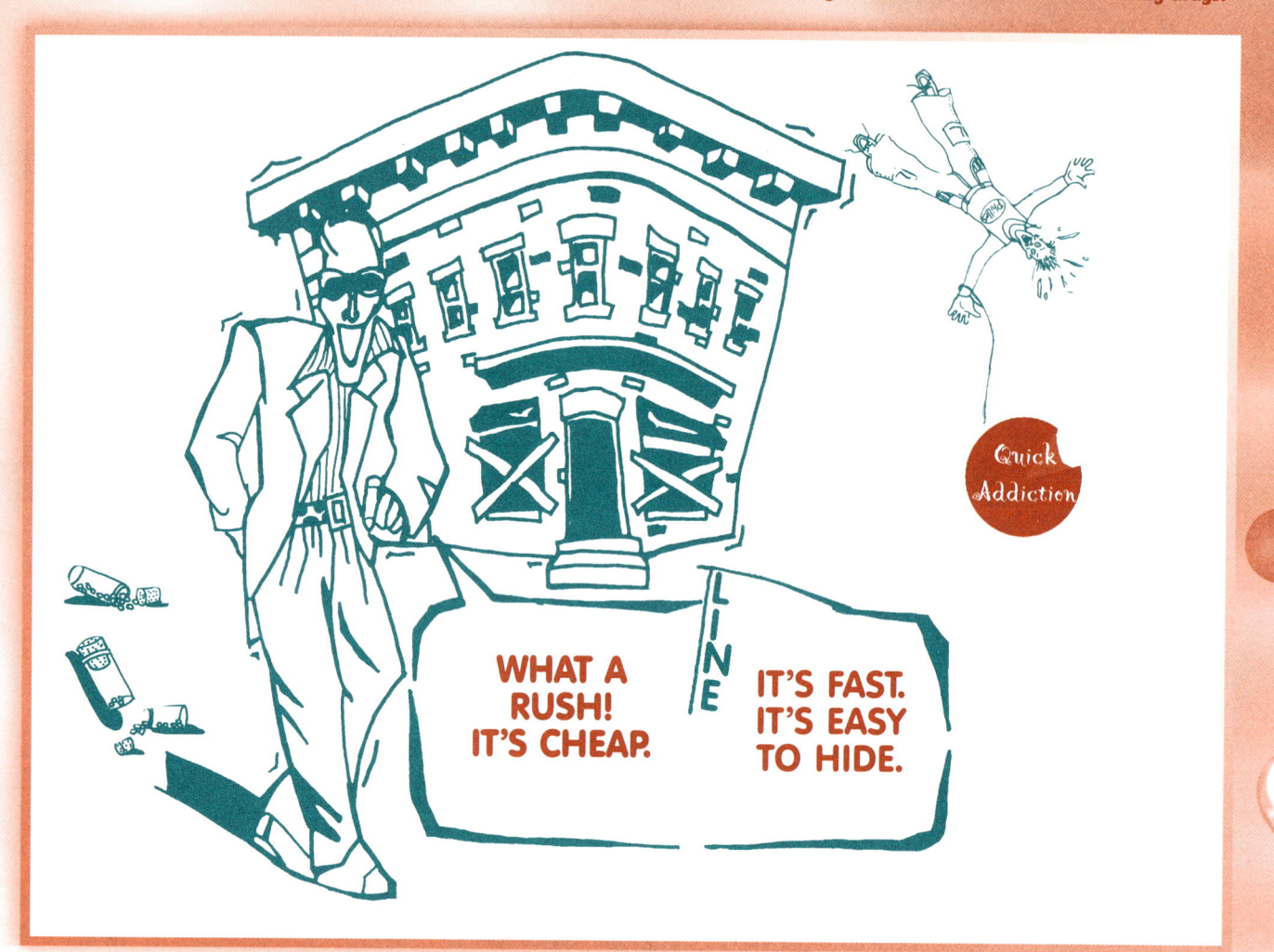

WHAT A RUSH! IT'S CHEAP.

IT'S FAST. IT'S EASY TO HIDE.

Quick Addiction

THINK ABOUT IT...

Use the cartoon above to answer the following questions:

HOOK — What drug is often sold in vials?

LINE — What attracts teens to this drug?

SINKER — What makes this drug particularly dangerous?

Be Street Smart

Stand up for what you know is right. Walk away from trouble!

For Advice and Information Call:

1-800-COCAINE
1-800-262-2463

68   CRACK   Street Smarts

CHECKUP

MATCHING

Column A   Column B

1. ___ binge   a. place where crack is sold and smoked
2. ___ crack   b. plastic container in which crack is sold
3. ___ vial   c. to use continually
4. ___ crash   d. cocaine that is smoked
5. ___ crack house e. intense "low"; feeling of depression

FILL IN THE BLANKS

addicted   money   sell   smoke
cocaine   '80s   rock

Crack is made from_____. It is also called _____. Crack began appearing in major cities in the _____.

Drug users _____ crack because it gives them a strong high feeling.

Drug dealers like crack because it is easy to _____. Users quickly become _____. Dealers then have a constant source of _____.

MULTIPLE CHOICE

1. **Crack is made from:**
   a. cocaine
   b. heroin
   c. marijuana

2. **Crack is also known as:**
   a. "rock"
   b. "weed"
   c. "pot"

3. **Crack**
   a. has medical uses
   b. does not have medical uses
   c. is a form of heroin

4. **Continual use of crack is called**
   a. binge
   b. insomnia
   c. depression

5. **The brain**
   a. is affected by crack
   b. is not affected by crack
   c. repels crack

TAKE A STAND

Dear Mrs. D.

IMPROVE YOUR REFUSAL SKILLS

Dear Mrs. D.:
My neighborhood may not be the classiest one, but it has always been clean and safe.
Two months ago, new owners bought the corner house. They put up a chain-link fence and bought two dobermans to patrol the yard. No one has ever met the new owners.
All sorts of people are in and out of that house, day and night. The driveway always has cars in it.
I hear rumors of the new "crack" house in our area and feel certain it's this house. What can I do?

Signed,
Scared silly

Write how you would answer if you were Mrs. D.

Mrs. D. Answers:
_____
_____
_____
_____
_____
_____
_____
_____
_____

Show that you recognize the danger by completing the exercise below.

Mike lives in what he called the "fake projects". He and his mom have a nice apartment with lots of space. Once inside, he feels safe, especially after his mom gets home from work at eight.
Outside he doesn't feel too good, but he tries to act like he isn't scared. He knows two apartments where crack is made. Some of his "friends" use crack and sell it to make extra money. They have been after him to hang out with them..

1. **Underline** two sentences that signal danger for Mike.

2. **Circle** a sentence that tells how Mike's family situation may make saying No to crack hard for Mike.

3. What positive plan can Mike have to stay safe and away from drug use? _____
_____
_____

Write the "coolest" way to say, "No!"

1. **The Offer** "Hey Sally, James gave me two vials of crack. Let's give it a try."
   You say _____
   _____

2. **The Dare** "So you drink a few beers and get buzzed, big deal! I bet you can't handle the rush that crack gives!"
   You say _____
   _____
   _____

3. **The Threat** "Jackie got us free samples of crack. EVERYONE has agreed to try it. Try it or you're out of the group."
   You say _____
   _____
   _____

4. **The Feel Good Approach** "I can see you're really down, a little crack and you won't remember feeling bad."
   You say: _____
   _____
   _____

BACK OFF

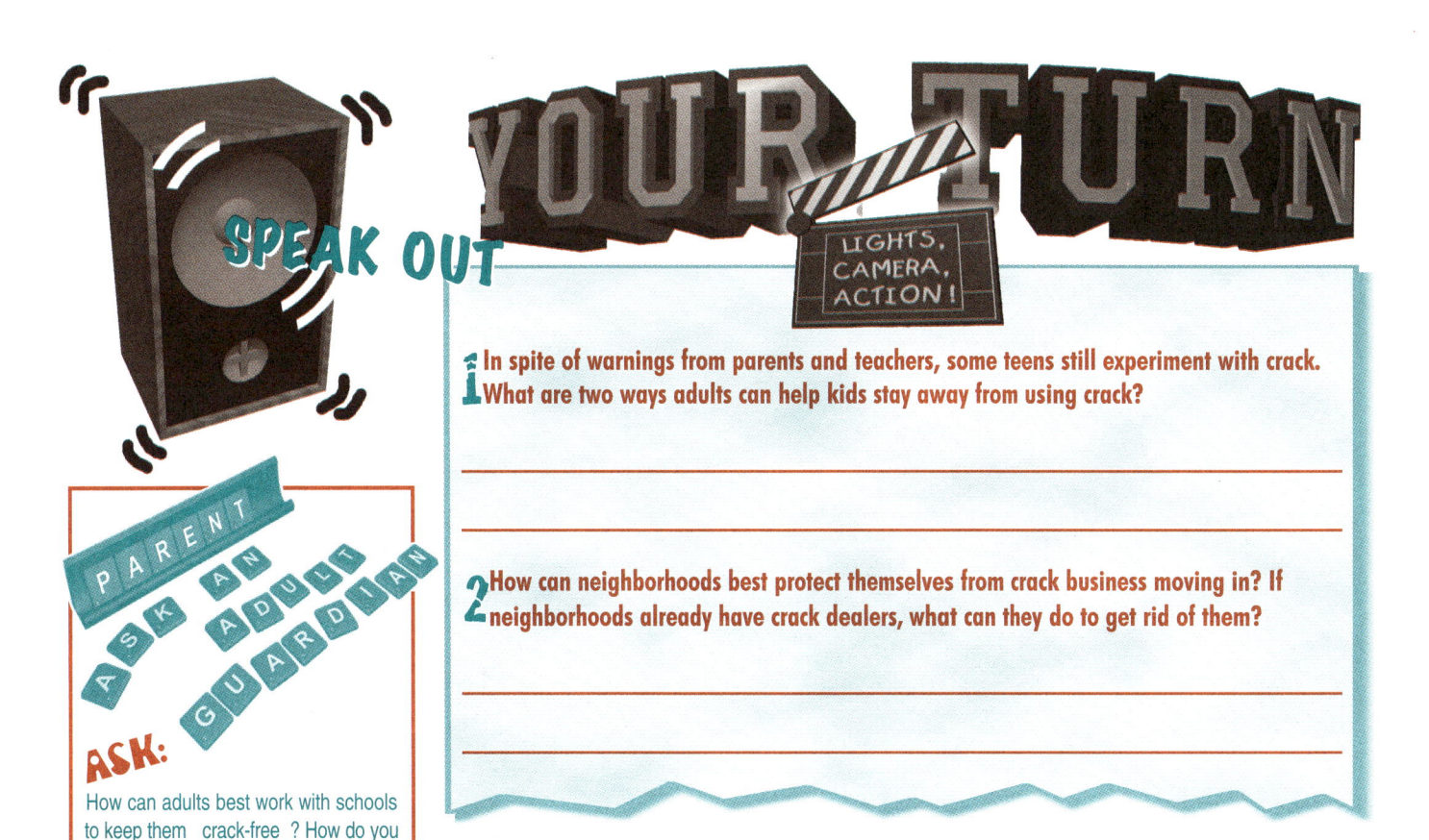

YOUR TURN

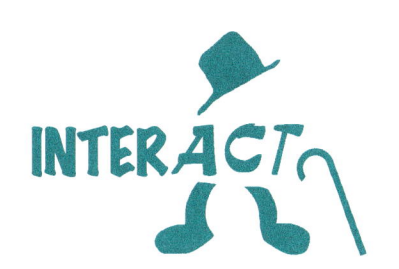

SPEAK OUT

LIGHTS, CAMERA, ACTION!

1. In spite of warnings from parents and teachers, some teens still experiment with crack. What are two ways adults can help kids stay away from using crack?

_____

_____

2. How can neighborhoods best protect themselves from crack business moving in? If neighborhoods already have crack dealers, what can they do to get rid of them?

_____

_____

ASK A PARENT AN ADULT GUARDIAN

ASK: How can adults best work with schools to keep them crack-free? How do you feel teens should protect themselves from teen drug dealers?

INTERACT

Setting: Between classes you go into the men's room. As you enter you see two kids exchanging money and small vials. One of the kids recognizes you and says, "Hey Eric, you didn't see anything. Remember that if you want to stay healthy."

Situation: You are scared but you don't like being threatened. You are also angry that these kind of kids are giving your school "a reputation." You also don't know what they might do.

Solution: Act out the way you would handle this situation. Have classmates role play the scene. Feel free to add any characters that might help you solve the problem.

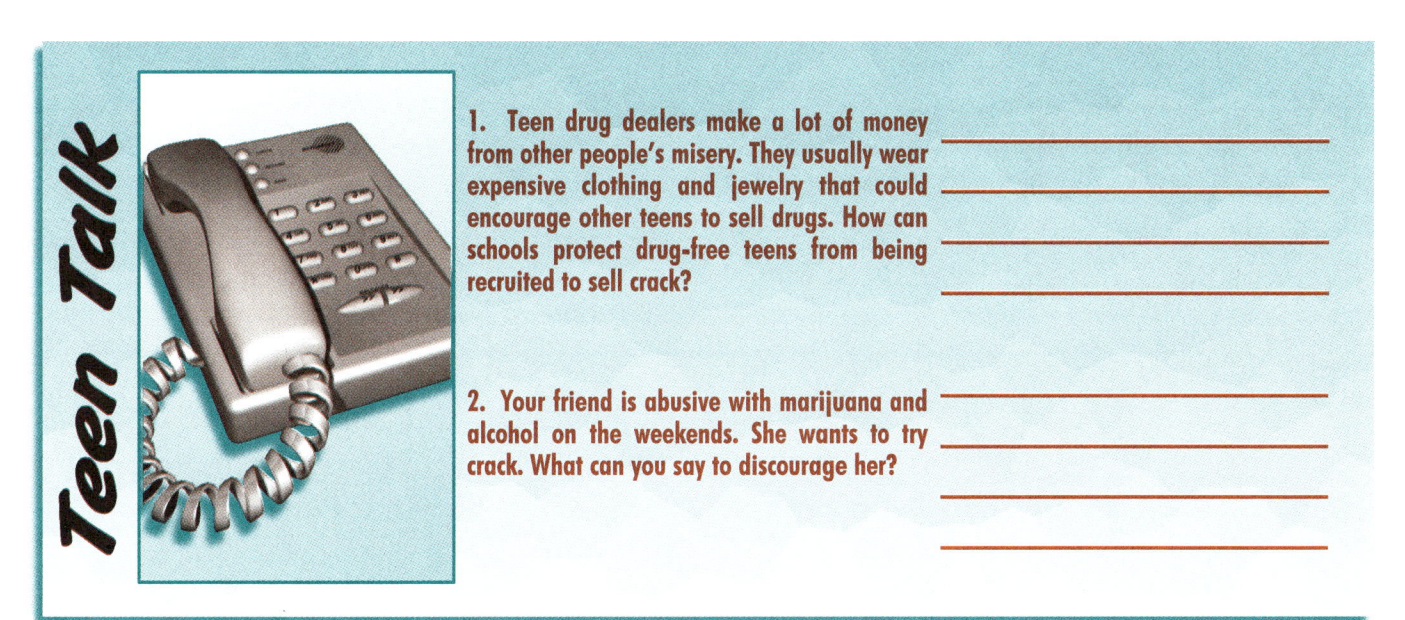

Teen Talk

1. Teen drug dealers make a lot of money from other people's misery. They usually wear expensive clothing and jewelry that could encourage other teens to sell drugs. How can schools protect drug-free teens from being recruited to sell crack?

_____

_____

2. Your friend is abusive with marijuana and alcohol on the weekends. She wants to try crack. What can you say to discourage her?

_____

_____

HEROIN CHAPTER 9

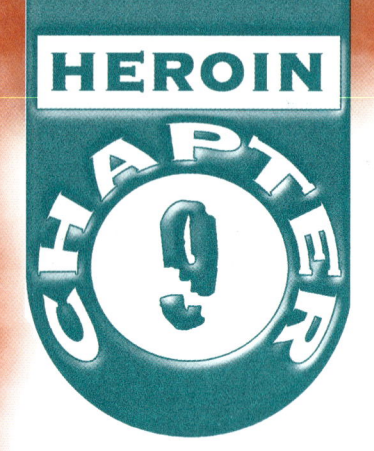

ON THE STREETS

"Hey, sister, what's up with you?" Jake said, blocking her way on the sidewalk.

Sharrie froze. Her heart was pounding. "Nothing. Let me be."

Jake moved in closer. "Okay. But it doesn't look like nothing. To me it looks like you're not feeling good, right? I watched you get off the bus this morning. I also saw you make that $10 heroin buy. This city is no place for a runaway with a habit. A pretty girl like you could get into a lot of trouble."

Sharrie tried to sound firm. "Go away. If you don't back off, I'm going to yell."

Jake's voice was calm. "You're going to yell! Who

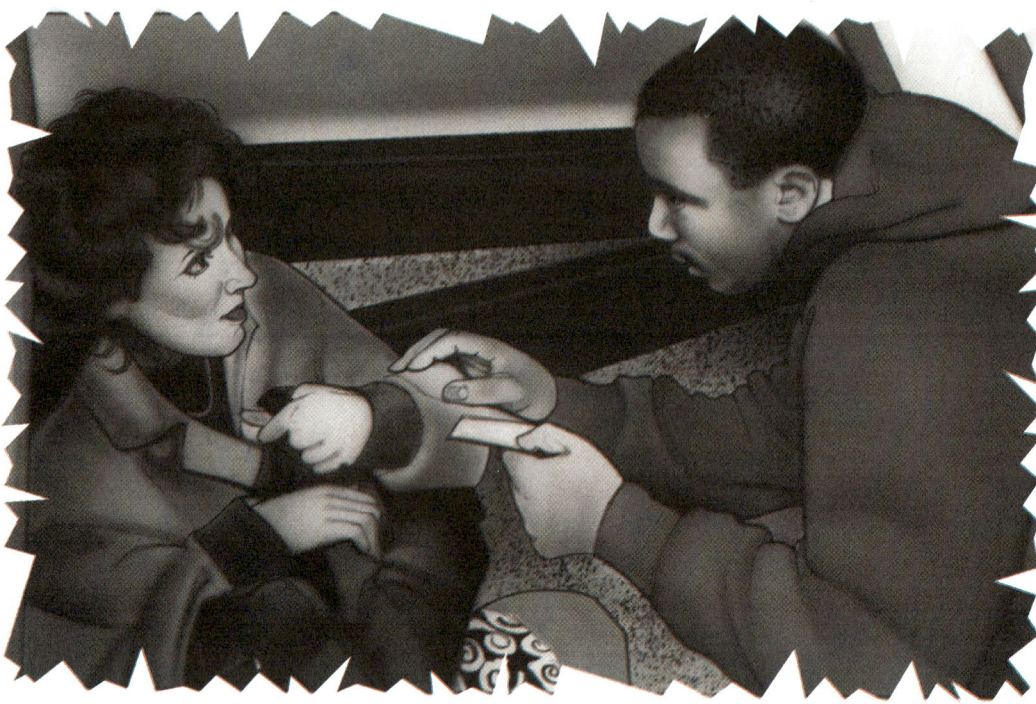

"I'M NO JUNKIE. JUST LEAVE ME ALONE!"

are you going to call? Your parents? The police?"

Sharrie's body was screaming to her for heroin. She was "strung out", angry and upset. She couldn't think straight and didn't know what to do or say.

Jake broke the silence with a laugh that almost sounded comforting. "Girl, I'm not the enemy. And I'm not trying to hit on you. I work for the drug rehab center. Part of my job is what we call 'last ditch rescue'. We try to..."

"Look, Mister, I don't know who you are and I don't care. I'm no junkie. Just leave me alone!"

Face Facts

Jake's eyes narrowed. His face lost its smile. He moved close to Sharrie and growled, "Listen up. I'm going to say this once. I saw you make the buy and I watched you snort it. It doesn't matter if you smoke heroin, inject it, snort it or eat it. Once it's got you, you're a junkie. I see dozens of kids like you. Most get off that bus like you, too proud or too stupid to go back home."

Jake continued, "In two months, life on the streets eats them up. They do whatever is necessary to get their supply. Nothing else matters. Thing is, they never go home, at least not alive. So run if you want, but face facts: either stop using now or forget about going back."

Sharrie crouched further into the corner. She had no answer.

Jake put his hand on her shoulder. "Look, in about two hours it will be dark. Then, the real "slimes" come out. You're going to be one terrified lady. The rehab center is just two blocks East. I can't make you come, but think about what will happen if you don't."

Jake pulled a card with his name, the center's address and phone number from his pocket, and handed it to Sharrie.

Homeward Bound

Jake continued, "Think about it. Why not come in and talk? You don't have to stay. We'll try to help you here, or find someone back home who will."

It was that card that had gotten her back home. Thanks to Jake, she was here with Sergeant Leguero and Mrs. D. ready to try to help herself.

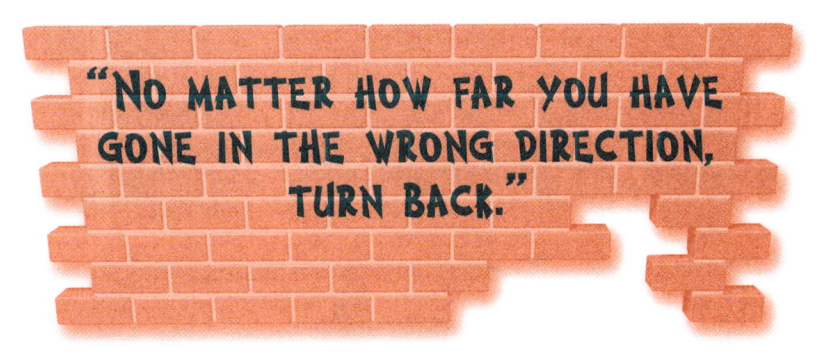

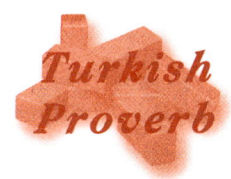

"NO MATTER HOW FAR YOU HAVE GONE IN THE WRONG DIRECTION, TURN BACK."

Turkish Proverb

TELL IT

H Is For Heroin, G Is For Greed

Heroin is known on the street as horse, smack and junk. It is made from the unripened seedpod of the opium poppy plant. It is grown in South Asia, South America and Central America. The poppy plant produces an illegal white or gray powder that is called heroin. It is very addictive.

Heroin is so addictive that few heroin abusers are able to quit their habit. This makes heroin sales very profitable. Powerful drug cartels organize criminal groups to control the illegal trade. Drug lords and street sellers protect their investment using guns and fear as weapons. To increase profits, drug dealers often cut or dilute the heroin with other street drugs, sugar, starch or even poison before selling it. The buyer can never be sure what they have bought. The ingredients and potency depend on what the dealers decide to sell.

Mainlining, Skin Popping And Snorting

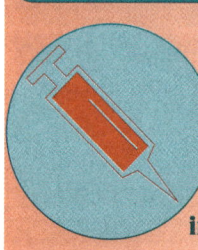

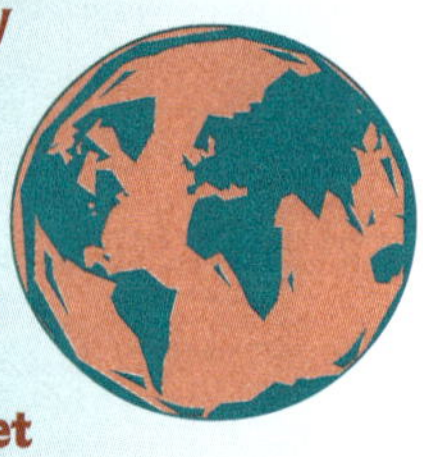

Heroin may be taken into the body in several ways. An abuser mainlines by injecting a mixture of dissolved, heated heroin and water into a vein. If an abuser skinpops heroin, it is injected just below the skin. Since stronger heroin and mixtures of heroin and synthetics are now available, some abusers snort or inhale heroin powder directly into their nose.

Too Young to Die

Easy access to heroin has made the drug available to a younger age group. Teens may be tempted to "snort" heroin at parties because they falsely believe that heroin is not dangerous if it is not injected. What these teens do not realize is that snorted heroin is often often 95% stronger. Also, "snorters" often become "mainliners" when they turn to injecting heroin in order to increase the effects.

Government officials are greatly alarmed by the increase in heroin related deaths. In addition to the dangers of the drug itself, there is also concern about the dangers to abusers and society as dealers fight for control of the market and their "turf" (territory).

Double Trouble

Often abusers who inject meet in "shooting galleries" to share drugs and needles. When I.V. drug needles are shared, small amounts of blood remain in the needle. The next user is getting heroin mixed with small amounts of someone else's blood! This exchange of blood and fluids increases the spread of the HIV/AIDs virus and hepatitis.

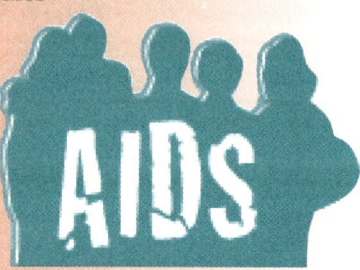

Abusers of crack/cocaine may snort heroin to lessen the severe "lows" of a coke crash. This often leads to cross addiction. The user is now addicted to two drugs instead of one.

STREET SMART STRATEGIES

KNOWLEDGE POWER: Learn about the dangers of heroin use.
CORE VALUES: Don't quit on yourself. Overcoming problems takes determination.
PROACTION: Take a stand — practice heroin refusal skills

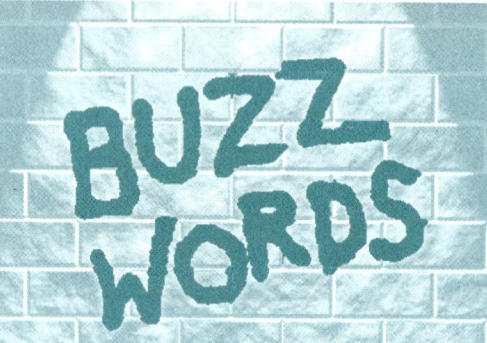

BUZZ WORDS

1. **Cartel** — an association of drug producers and sellers that set prices and control the drug market
2. **Drug lord** — most powerful person who controls the drug business
3. **Dual or cross-addiction** — to be addicted to more than one drug
4. **Endorphin** — natural chemical produced by the body, allows person to feel natural highs and lows
5. **Hepatitis** — a liver disease spread through the exchange of blood
6. **Heroin** — (*horse, smack, junk*) is highly addictive drug made from the seeds of the poppy plant
7. **Mainline** — to inject heroin directly into a vein with a needle
8. **Methadone** — legal, man-made addictive drug sometimes used in the treatment of heroin addicts
9. **Potency** — strength of a drug
10. **Seedpod** — part of plant that holds and protects the seeds
11. **Shooting gallery** — place where abusers go to inject themselves with heroin
12. **Skinpop** — to inject heroin under the surface of skin
13. **Snorting** — inhaling heroin through the nose
14. **STD** — sexually transmitted disease
15. **Synthetics** — not naturally occuring, made of chemicals
16. **Tolerance** — the increasing need for greater amounts of a drug in order to feel the original "high" feeling
17. **Withdrawal** — powerful symptoms that occur when abuser stops using drug; pain, vomiting, convulsions

Show It

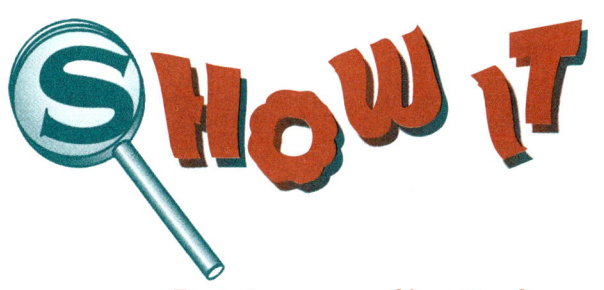

THE HEROIN HIGH

First time users of heroin often get nauseous because the body is rejecting a poisonous substance. Continued use may result in a sense of warmth and "well-being" which lasts about eight to ten hours. As the heroin wears off, the person feels depressed. To regain that feeling of well-being, more of the drug is needed. This increased demand is known as tolerance. The tolerance level continually increases causing a need for more heroin. This often leads the abuser to some type of criminal activity to pay for the habit.

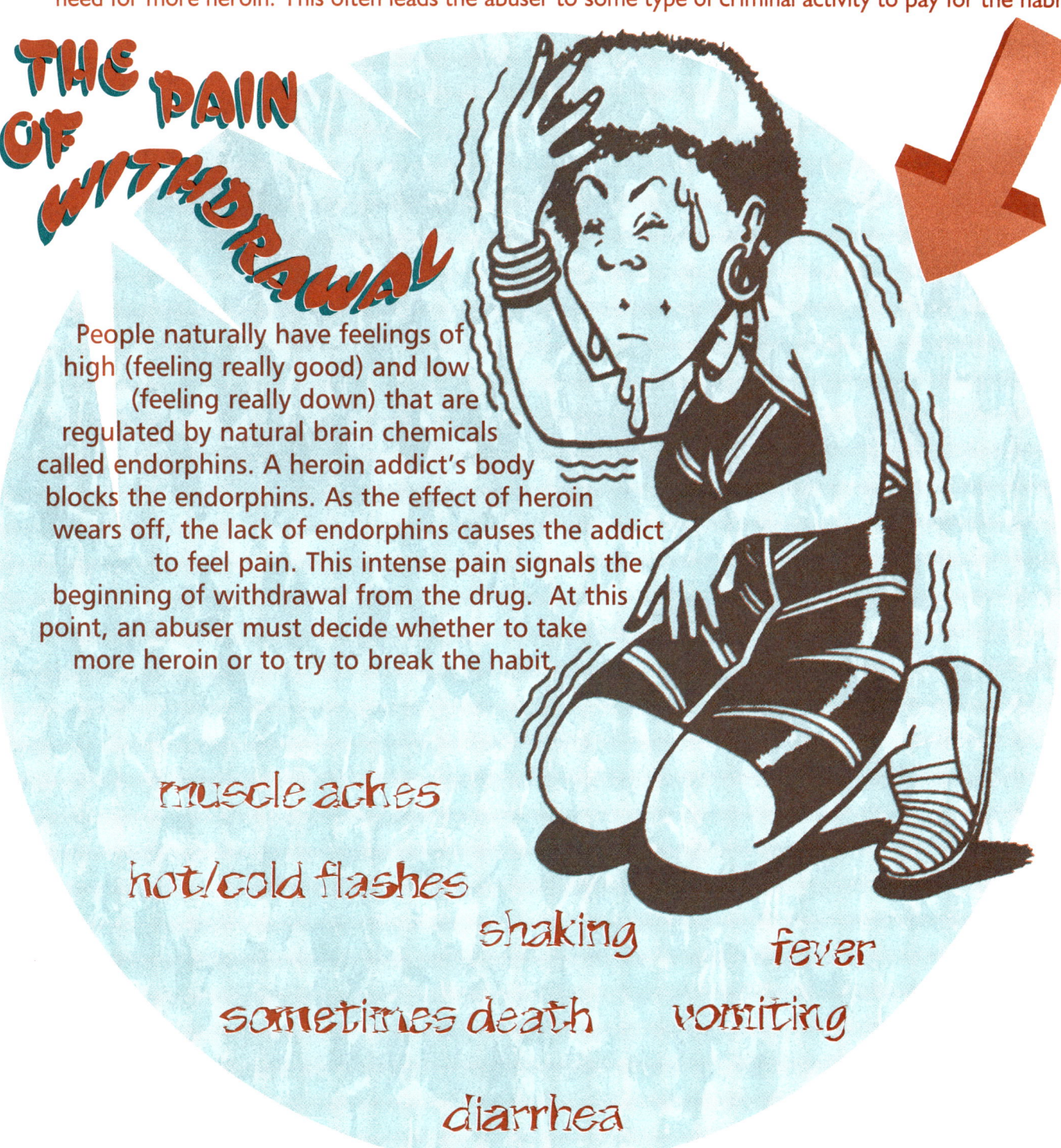

THE PAIN OF WITHDRAWAL

People naturally have feelings of high (feeling really good) and low (feeling really down) that are regulated by natural brain chemicals called endorphins. A heroin addict's body blocks the endorphins. As the effect of heroin wears off, the lack of endorphins causes the addict to feel pain. This intense pain signals the beginning of withdrawal from the drug. At this point, an abuser must decide whether to take more heroin or to try to break the habit.

- muscle aches
- hot/cold flashes
- shaking
- fever
- sometimes death
- vomiting
- diarrhea

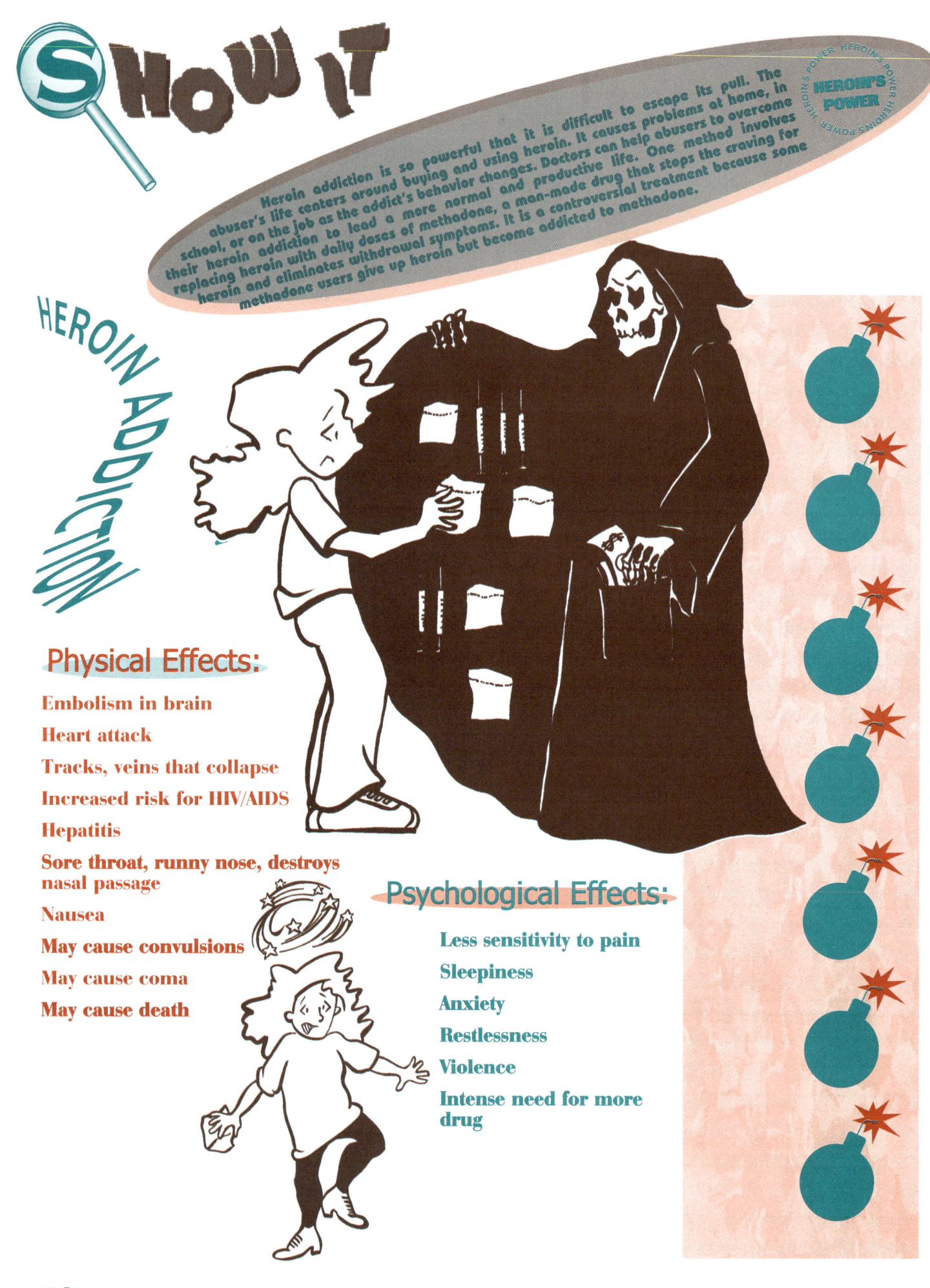

SHOW IT

HEROIN ADDICTION

HEROIN'S POWER

Heroin addiction is so powerful that it is difficult to escape its pull. The abuser's life centers around buying and using heroin. It causes problems at home, in school, or on the job as the addict's behavior changes. Doctors can help abusers to overcome their heroin addiction to lead a more normal and productive life. One method involves replacing heroin with daily doses of methadone, a man-made drug that stops the craving for heroin and eliminates withdrawal symptoms. It is a controversial treatment because some methadone users give up heroin but become addicted to methadone.

Physical Effects:

Embolism in brain

Heart attack

Tracks, veins that collapse

Increased risk for HIV/AIDS

Hepatitis

Sore throat, runny nose, destroys nasal passage

Nausea

May cause convulsions

May cause coma

May cause death

Psychological Effects:

Less sensitivity to pain

Sleepiness

Anxiety

Restlessness

Violence

Intense need for more drug

HEROIN

Street Smarts

HOOK, LINE, AND SINKER

HOOK: The drugs that get people hooked. **LINE:** The lie that gets them to take the drugs. **SINKER:** The bad results of taking drugs.

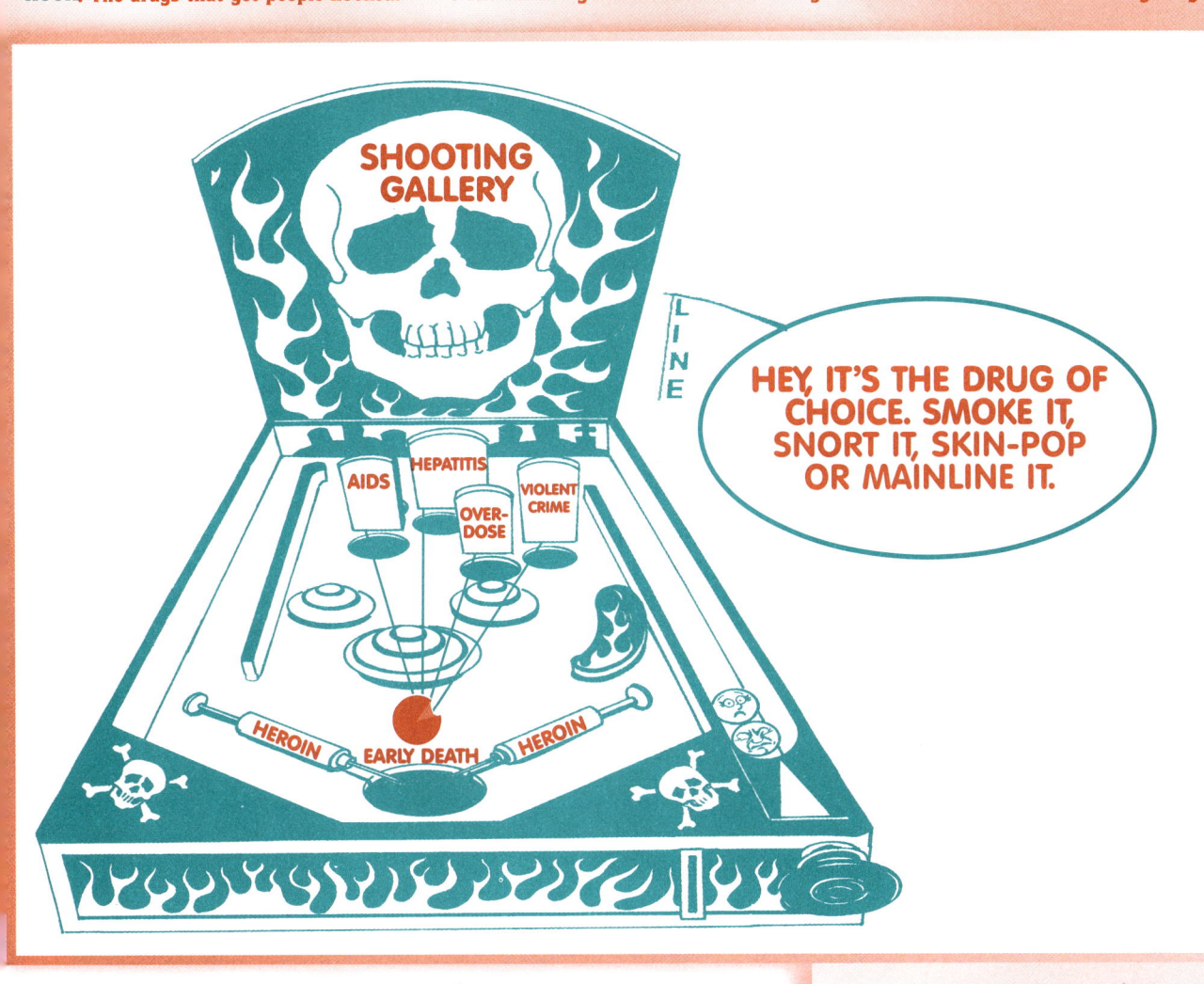

SHOOTING GALLERY

Labels on pinball machine: AIDS, HEPATITIS, OVERDOSE, VIOLENT CRIME, HEROIN, EARLY DEATH, HEROIN

LINE: HEY, IT'S THE DRUG OF CHOICE. SMOKE IT, SNORT IT, SKIN-POP OR MAINLINE IT.

THINK ABOUT IT...

Use the cartoon above to answer the following questions:

HOOK — Which drug is often abused in shooting galleries?

LINE — How are teens tempted to try this drug?

SINKER — What may result from an overdose?

Be Street Smart

Heroin users are at increased risk for HIV/AIDS.

Choose your friends wisely!

For Advice And Information Call:

National Council on Alcoholism and Drug Dependence (NCADD)

1-800-NCA-Call
or
http://www.ncadd.org

THE PEOPLES PUBLISHING GROUP, 1-800-822-1080. COPYING PROHIBITED BY LAW.

CHECKUP

MATCHING

Column A	Column B
1. snort	a. secretly taken into a country
2. tolerance	b. inhale through the nose
3. endorphin	c. taking such a large amount of drug that it could kill
4. smuggled	d. having to take a larger dose of a drug in order to get the same effect.
5. overdose	e. the natural pain-reducing chemical made by the body

FILL IN THE BLANKS

Asia   painful   noses
withdrawal   skin popping   South America
dangerous   addictive   Central America

Heroin is an _____ drug. It is smuggled into our country from Southern_____ , _____ and _____. When heroin addicts inject the drug into a vein, it is called_____. When they inject it below the surface of the skin it is called_____. Recently, as heroin powder has become stronger, some abusers are snorting heroin through their_____. Any way that heroin is taken can be_____. When an addicted person stops taking heroin, their body goes through _____. Withdrawal is very _____. Close medical attention is needed.

MULTIPLE CHOICE

1. **Poppy plants grow**
   a. in North America and Alaska
   b. in Northern Europe and Africa
   c. in South and Central America and South Asia

2. **This man-made drug is sometimes prescribed to heroin abusers by doctors**
   a. smack
   b. methadone
   c. horse

3. **What happens when heroin is cut?**
   a. the amount becomes smaller
   b. the drug becomes stronger
   c. the drug is mixed with other substances

4. **A place where heroin abusers meet to share drugs and needles is called**
   a. a shooting gallery
   b. a cartel
   c. mainlining

5. **When drug abusers use more than one drug, they are**
   a. snorting
   b. skinpopping
   c. cross-addicted

HEROIN   Street Smarts

TAKE A STAND

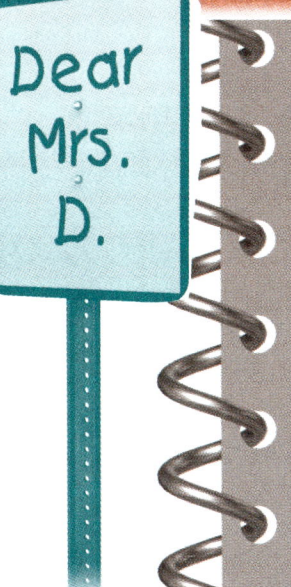

Dear Mrs. D.

IMPROVE YOUR REFUSAL SKILLS

Dear Mrs. D.:
 I'm worried about my best friend Rob. For the past two months he has been hanging out with a bunch of "druggies." His grades have fallen, but he doesn't care.
 Rob and I grew up together and I know he is really in over his head. He told me he was just going to try a little heroin, but now he's hooked.
 Our parents have been friends for a long time too. In a way I'd like to talk with his parents, but I don't know what to say.
 The truth is that I'm scared for him and angry that I've lost my best friend.

 Signed,
 Want to Help, But How?

Write how you would answer if you were Mrs. D.

Mrs. D. answers:
_____
_____
_____
_____
_____
_____
_____
_____
_____

Show that you recognize the danger by completing the exercise below.

DANGER

The housing project in which Ron and Jamie live is clean and safe. But the building next to it has drug pushers and users who hassle everyone who passes by. Ron and Jamie always try to avoid the other building.

Yesterday, as they ran through the yard behind both buildings, Jamie spotted a shopping cart filled with paper bags. When the boys went to investigate, they found that the paper bags were filled with small, plastic bags of fine white powder.

The boys believe the white powder in the plastic bags is heroin. They also know if it is heroin it is worth a lot of money.

1. <u>Underline</u> a sentence that shows how Ron and Jamie tried to avoid trouble.

2. (Circle) a sentence that tells what the boys suspect is in the plastic bags.

3. Who could the boys call about their find to avoid trouble?_____
_____

Write the "coolest" way to say, "No!"

1. **The Offer** "Hey, Juan, I found some 'smack'. Let's try it."

   You say _____
   _____
   _____

2. **The Dare** "Listen, John, if you want to hang with the posse, you've got to shoot some 'horse'."

   You say _____
   _____
   _____

   BACK OFF

3. **The Threat** "If you don't 'mainline' with us, Latoya, we're taking you home."

   You say _____
   _____
   _____

4. *The Feel Good Approach* "Go ahead and 'skin pop.' There's no feeling like it in the world."

   You say _____
   _____
   _____

YOUR TURN

SPEAK OUT

1. Heroin users often share I.V. needles. Why are they at increased risk of becoming HIV positive?

_____
_____

2. Why do many heroin users become cross-addicted?

_____
_____
_____

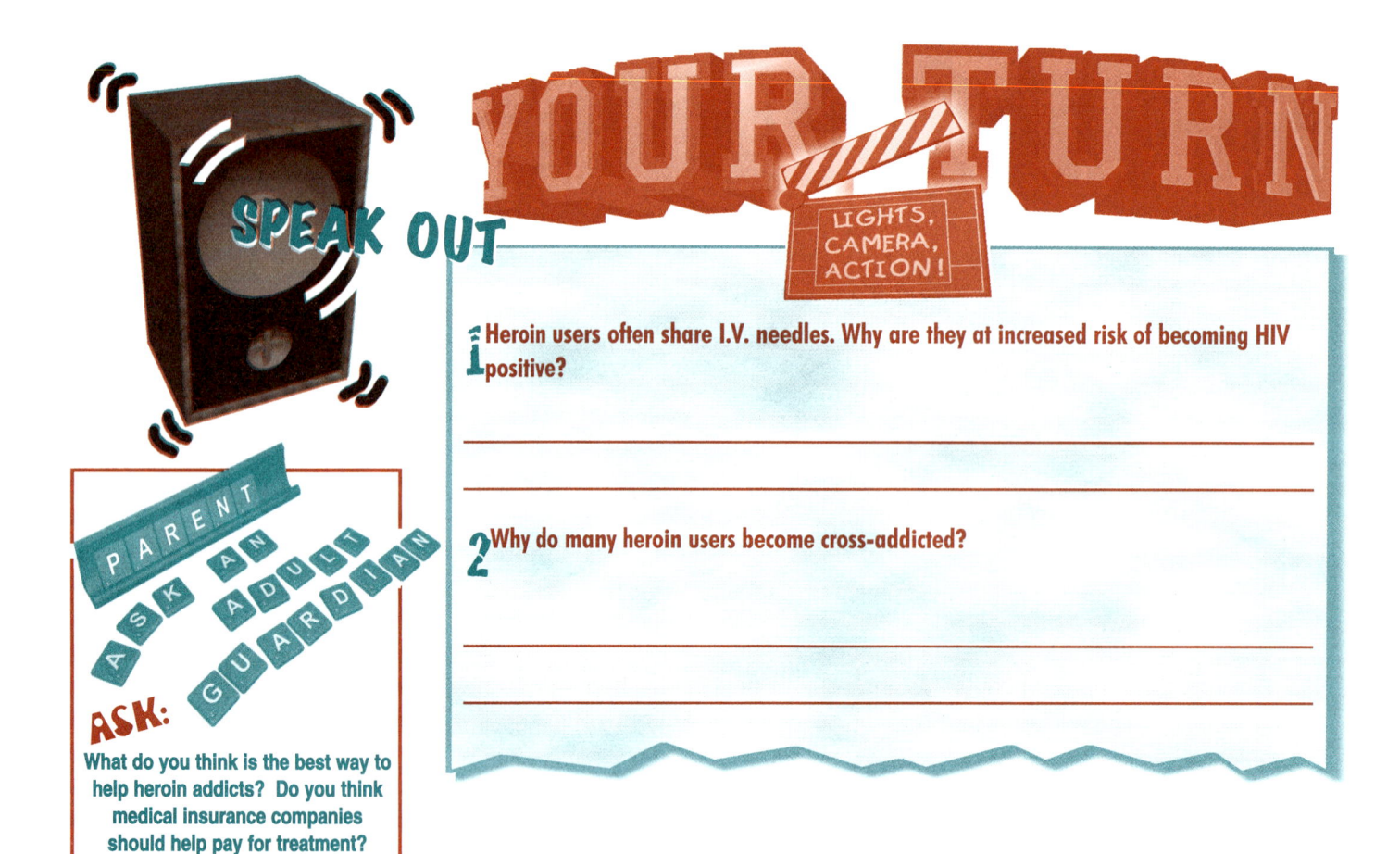

ASK A PARENT AN ADULT GUARDIAN

ASK: What do you think is the best way to help heroin addicts? Do you think medical insurance companies should help pay for treatment?

INTERACT

Setting: You are the parent of an 18-year-old senior. While cleaning his room, you accidentally knock the top off a shoe box in his closet. Inside you find equipment for I.V. drug use.

Situation: Your son has been acting strange for the last two months. Every time you try to talk to him, he doesn't pay attention.

Solution: Act out the scene between you and your son. Remember that your first concern is to get him help.

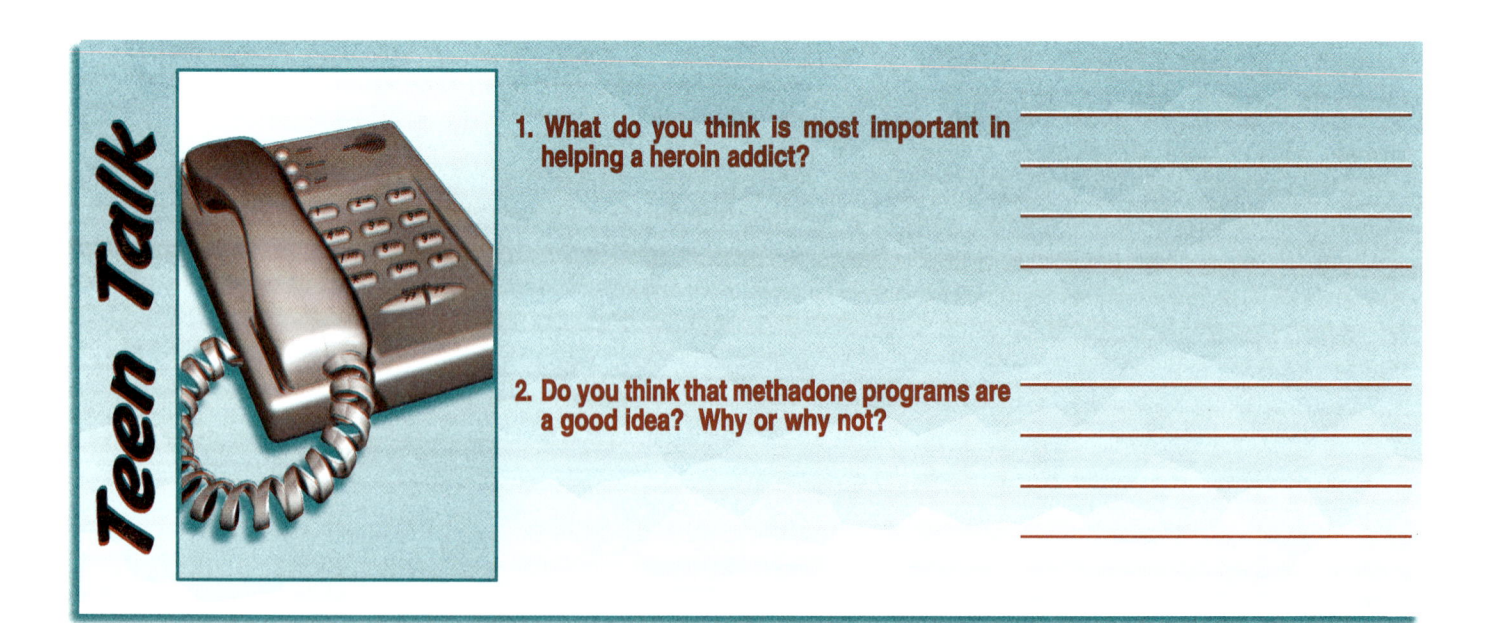

Teen Talk

1. What do you think is most important in helping a heroin addict?

_____
_____
_____
_____

2. Do you think that methadone programs are a good idea? Why or why not?

_____
_____
_____
_____

AMPHETAMINES DEPRESSANTS

CHAPTER 10

THE HOME-COMING QUEEN

The "No-Mores" had agreed that Leguero's idea to help the students in Central High's drug program stay clean was worth doing. But now that the big day was here, they weren't sure they wanted to do it.

A few of the "No-Mores" were former students. Some were afraid of going back and facing their peers, but as Sergeant Leguero pointed out, they really had little choice. Community service was part of the "sentence" the judge had handed down to get them involved in giving something positive back to the community.

So here they were at Central High School to encourage students to admit to their drug problem and take steps to become drug-free.

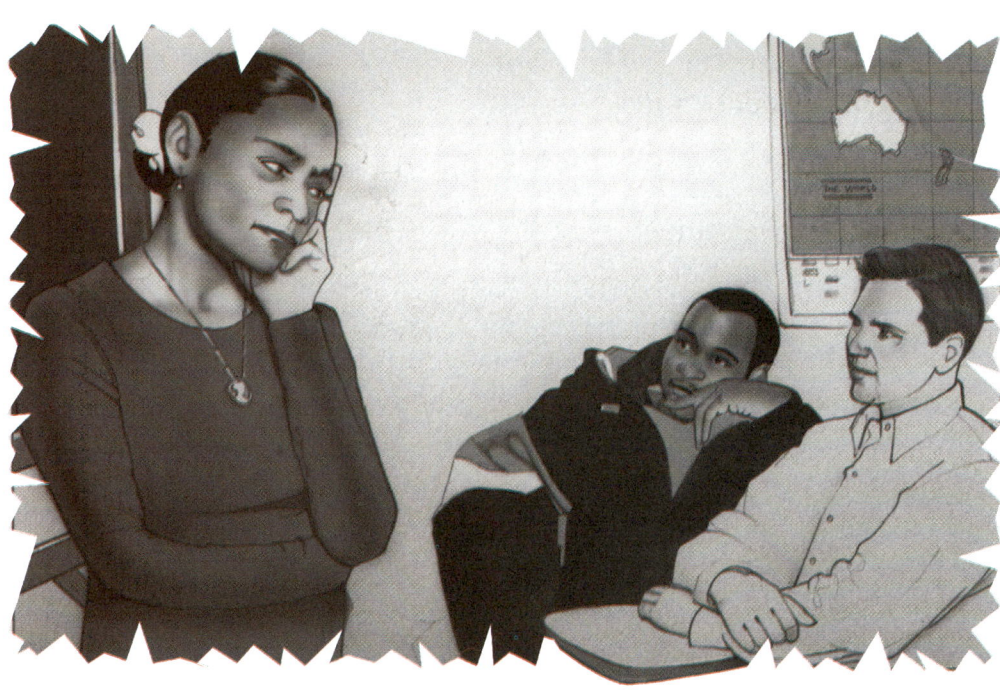

"I knew better but I didn't consider the consequences."

Some of the kids from Central were curious about the "No-Mores" since quite a few of them had been expelled or had dropped out of school. Had these kids really changed? Could they really help with someone else's drug problem?

In the Spotlight

Sandy stood nervously in the speaker's spot. She knew she could con Mr. Adams, the drug counselor. She knew she couldn't fool the "No-Mores." They had seen and done everything. She thought about all the times she had called them "druggies" and losers. She remembered making fun of "those low lifes." Now she was one of them. A mocking voice broke through her thoughts.

"Kind of a come-down, isn't it? Miss Sandy Homecoming Queen is going to address us. Let's hear it for Miss All-American Speed Freak!" Carlos said loudly.

"The guys whistled and clapped. Sergeant Leguero was embarrassed. He had brought the "No-Mores" here to help, not to put anyone down. Before Leguero could speak, Sandy cut him off.

"Who are you to talk, Carlos? I hear that since your last LSD trip, your mother has to dress you."

Leguero's firm voice cut the group's laughter short. "Carlos, you deserved that. Your remarks were uncalled for. Give Sandy a chance."

Sandy sent Leguero a look of appreciation. She took a deep breath and began.

"Ever since grade school kids have told me how lucky I am. I had lots of friends and no problems at school. The honor roll wasn't hard for me. And I loved being captain of the gymnastic team."

"But when I got to Central, there was more competition. Part of me enjoyed it, the other part of me was frightened I wouldn't measure up any more. I had to work harder. I guess I was used to being the best and was afraid of anything less."

"I can't blame anyone for what happened. I knew better but didn't consider the consequences. I felt really stressed. I started taking pills to give me that extra push to study for exams. When my grades started to slip, it never dawned on me that it was because I couldn't concentrate. I took more pills so I could study more. On weekends I felt wiped out. I couldn't even enjoy games or parties."

Losing Control

Carlos was surprised to hear Sandy admit that everything didn't come so easy to her. Instead of making fun of her, he was beginning to understand. Calling out once more, he said, "Hey, that's rough when sports and parties are no fun!"

Sandy felt more comfortable as she sensed the group's acceptance. "Yea, that's why I started taking the sleeping pills. I knew I needed to get some rest, so I borrowed some pills my mom had gotten from her doctor. But it didn't really help.

"Things were out of control. During the week, uppers, weekends, downers. I was moody and irritable. I figured it was because I was always working. So when the kids pushed me to go to the Halloween party, I did."

"I was so exhausted, I popped a few uppers before the party so I could be a part of the fun. Then once I got to the party, I wanted to relax so I had a few beers: that was my ticket to the emergency room. It's not pleasant having your stomach pumped. It's not pleasant realizing you might have ended your own life."

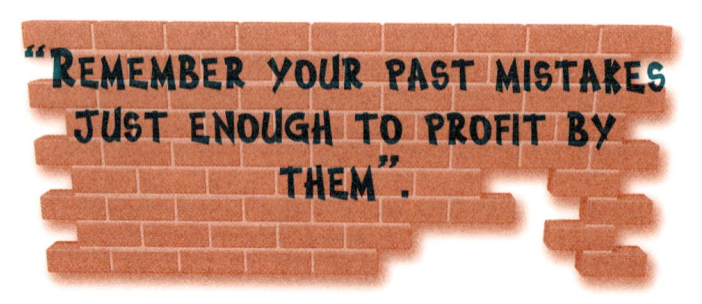

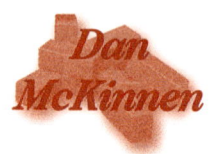

"REMEMBER YOUR PAST MISTAKES JUST ENOUGH TO PROFIT BY THEM".

Dan McKinnen

TELL IT

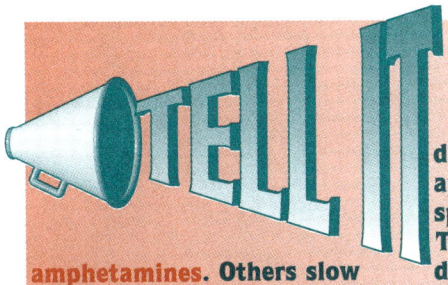

Up And Down

There are many man-made drugs that affect our minds and bodies. Some drugs speed up body functions. These drugs are called **amphetamines**. Others slow down the body's responses. These drugs are known as **depressants**.

Amphetamines and depressants have legal forms that can be prescribed by doctors and used as medicines. There are also forms that are prepared illegally and sold on the streets.

Racing Into Trouble

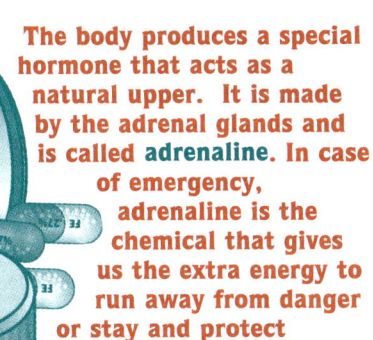

The body produces a special hormone that acts as a natural upper. It is made by the adrenal glands and is called **adrenaline**. In case of emergency, adrenaline is the chemical that gives us the extra energy to run away from danger or stay and protect ourselves.

Amphetamines are man-made pills that stimulate or "speed up" activities in the brain and nervous system. They are referred to as **uppers** because of their effect on the body. When amphetamines are taken, they cause a signal to be sent to the adrenal glands to release extra adrenaline into the bloodstream. Amphetamines cause the unnatural release of adrenaline for long periods of time. People who abuse amphetamines put great stress on their body. Abusers run the risk of damaging blood vessels that can result in heart and brain damage, stroke, or death.

Methamphetamines are illegal forms of amphetamines. Crank and ice are street names for two of them. Both are very dangerous. They are inexpensive to make, and are sold cheaply. They are very powerful and very addictive. They may cause violent aggressive behavior that sometimes lasts years after abuse has stopped.

Slow And Deadly

Drugs that affect mood and behavior by slowing down activities of the brain are called **depressants** or **downers**. **Barbiturates** are a type of depressant that doctors sometimes prescribe to help people sleep. Barbiturates are also known as "solid alcohol" because of its drunk-like effect. When taken for a continued period of time, tolerance develops. The user needs more of the drug to get the same effect. In time, the drug may lose its ability to cause the person to sleep.

Tranquilizers are another type of depressant. They may be prescribed by doctors to help people relax and calm down. Tranquilizers prescribed by a doctor are taken in small dosage. They can relieve tension and relax muscles. Illegal tranquilizers, taken in large doses, can cause coma or death.

STREET SMART STRATEGIES

KNOWLEDGE POWER: Learn about the dangers of amphetamine and depressant abuse.
CORE VALUES: Stress is natural. Deal with it naturally—exercise, meditate, read.
PROACTION: Take a stand—practice refusal skills for improper use of amphetamine and depressant drugs.

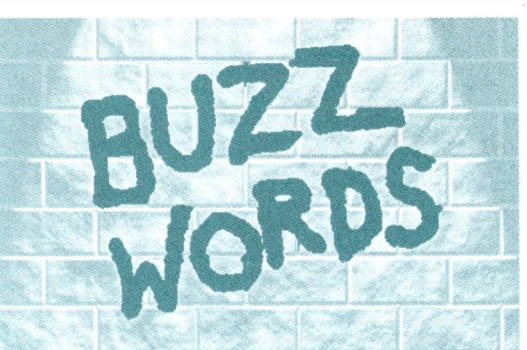

BUZZ WORDS

1. **Adrenaline** — hormone produced by adrenal glands that gives extra energy
2. **Amphetamines** — (*street name bennies, dexies*) stimulate or speed up body functions
3. **Barbiturates** — drugs that depress or slow down body functions
4. **Depressant** — drugs that slow down body functions
5. **Downers** — depressants, drugs that slow down body functions
6. **Dual addiction** — dependent upon two drugs; amphetamines for an "up," depressants for a "down"
7. **Ecstasy** — street name for illegal amphetamine type drug
8. **Infertile** — unable to have children
9. **Methamphetamines** — (*street name crank, ice, ecstasy*) is an illegal amphetamine-type drug
9. **Snort** — to take drug by sniffing, inhaling
10. **Tolerance** — body requires more drugs to get previous effect
11. **Tranquilizer** — depressant drug that slows down body functions
12. **Uppers** — amphetamine drugs that speed up body functions
14. **Runs** — repeated or continual drug use to avoid the "crash"

SHOW IT

When a person is hooked on two drugs at the same time, it is called dual addiction. Anyone with a dual addiction has doubled the danger to their health since their body must respond to the effects of *both* drugs. Persons who use amphetamines to give them extra energy sometimes have difficulty calming down. If a depressant is used to slow down body functions in order to relax or sleep it can result in dual addiction. This drug cycle causes a roller-coaster effect that is extremely dangerous.

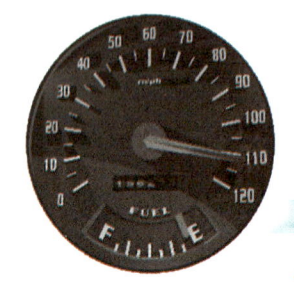

DOUBLE TROUBLE

AMPHETAMINE SPEEDING

Amphetamines have four basic strengths depending on how they are made.

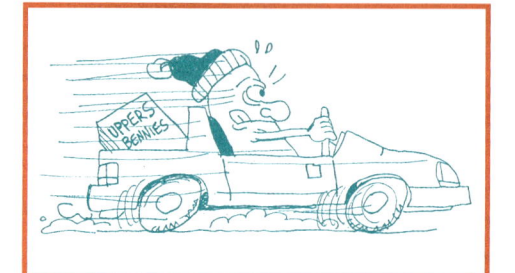

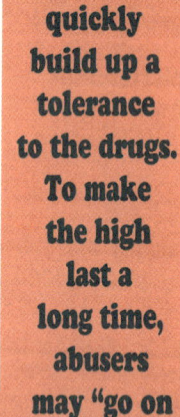

Amphetamine abusers quickly build up a tolerance to the drugs. To make the high last a long time, abusers may "go on a run". When an abuser "runs", amphetamines are taken every few hours for several days without food or sleep. When the drug finally wears off, the abuser may sleep for 24 hours without waking.

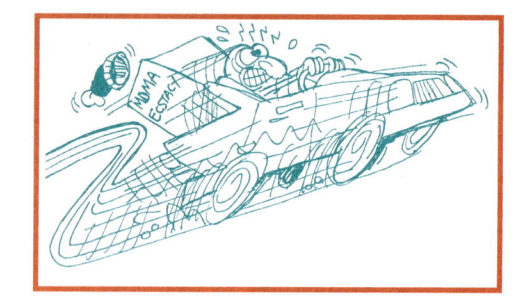

DRUG (Street Name)
Levoamphetamine (*uppers, bennies*)

METHOD USED
Tablets, snorted

STRENGTH
Varies, like "overdrive" in car

DRUG (Street Name)
Dextoamphetamine (*dexies, go-fast*)

METHOD USED
Tablets, snorted

STRENGTH
Fast, twice as powerful as uppers

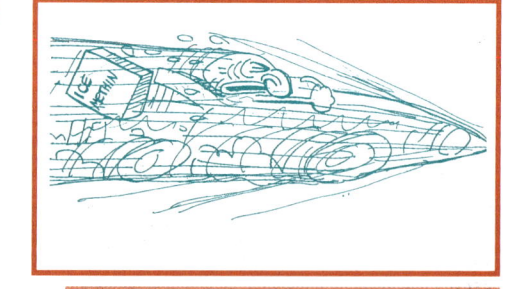

DRUG (Street Name)
Methylene-dioxy-methamphetamine (MDMA) (*ecstacy, love bug*)

METHOD USED
Pills, injected, snorted

STRENGTH
"Out of control," may cause halllucinations. Abusers see/hear things that are not real

DRUG (Street Name)
Methamphetamine (*ice, crank*)

METHOD USED
Smoked

STRENGTH
"Warp Speed", twice as powerful as dexies, lasts 60 times longer than crack

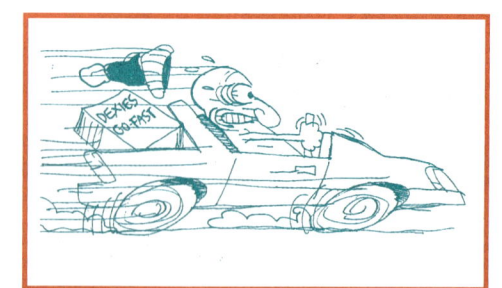

84   AMPHETAMINES/DEPRESSANTS   Street Smarts

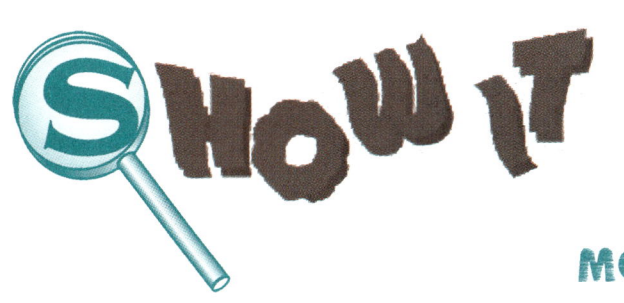

Show It

EFFECTS OF AMPHETAMINE ABUSE

PHYSICAL EFFECTS:

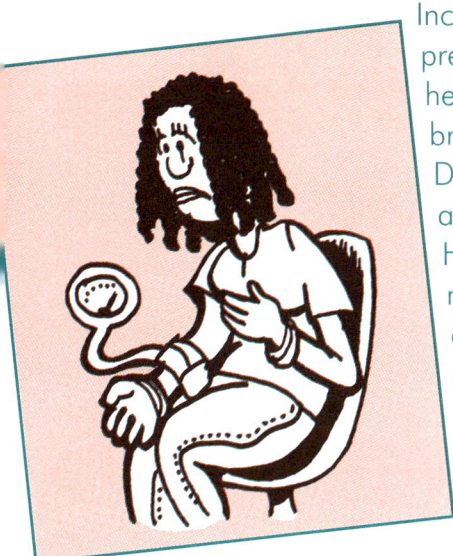

Increased blood pressure, heartbeat, breathing rate. Decreased appetite. Headaches, nausea, chills, dizziness. Female abusers may become infertile. Pregnant abusers often give birth to babies with birth defects.

MENTAL EFFECTS:

Abusers often "crash" when the effects of the drug wear off. "Crashing" causes depression. Such reactions as over-tiredness, inability to sleep, outbursts of temper or panic are not unusual. Some abusers hallucinate and have great feelings of anxiety. They may believe that "people are out to get them."

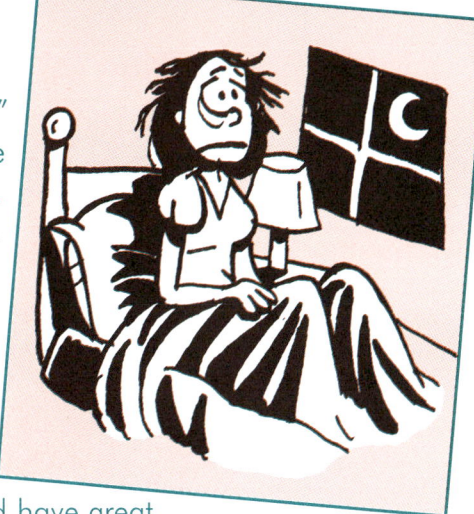

TRUTH ABOUT DEPRESSANTS

Only a medical doctor is qualified to prescribe tranquilizers or barbiturates. Doctors may prescribe them to relieve stress or help a person sleep. However, neither tranquilizers nor barbiturates solve the problem causing the stress. When abused, tranquilizers and barbiturates are highly addictive. When mixed with alcohol or other depressants, their effects are multiplied. Mixing can cause coma or death.

TRANQUILIZERS

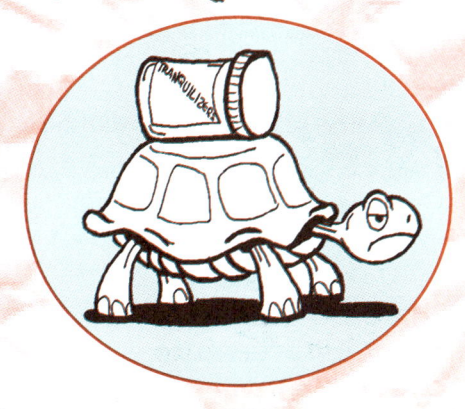

EFFECT
Help people to relax.

BARBITURATES

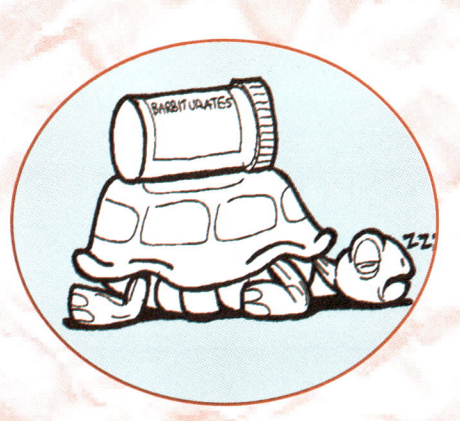

EFFECT
Causes sleep.

BARBITURATES, TRANQUILIZERS & ALCOHOL

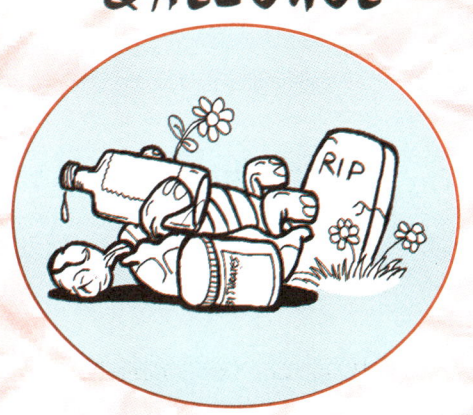

EFFECT
Death.

HOOK, LINE, AND SINKER

HOOK: The drugs that get people hooked. **LINE:** The lie that gets them to take the drugs. **SINKER:** The bad results of taking drugs.

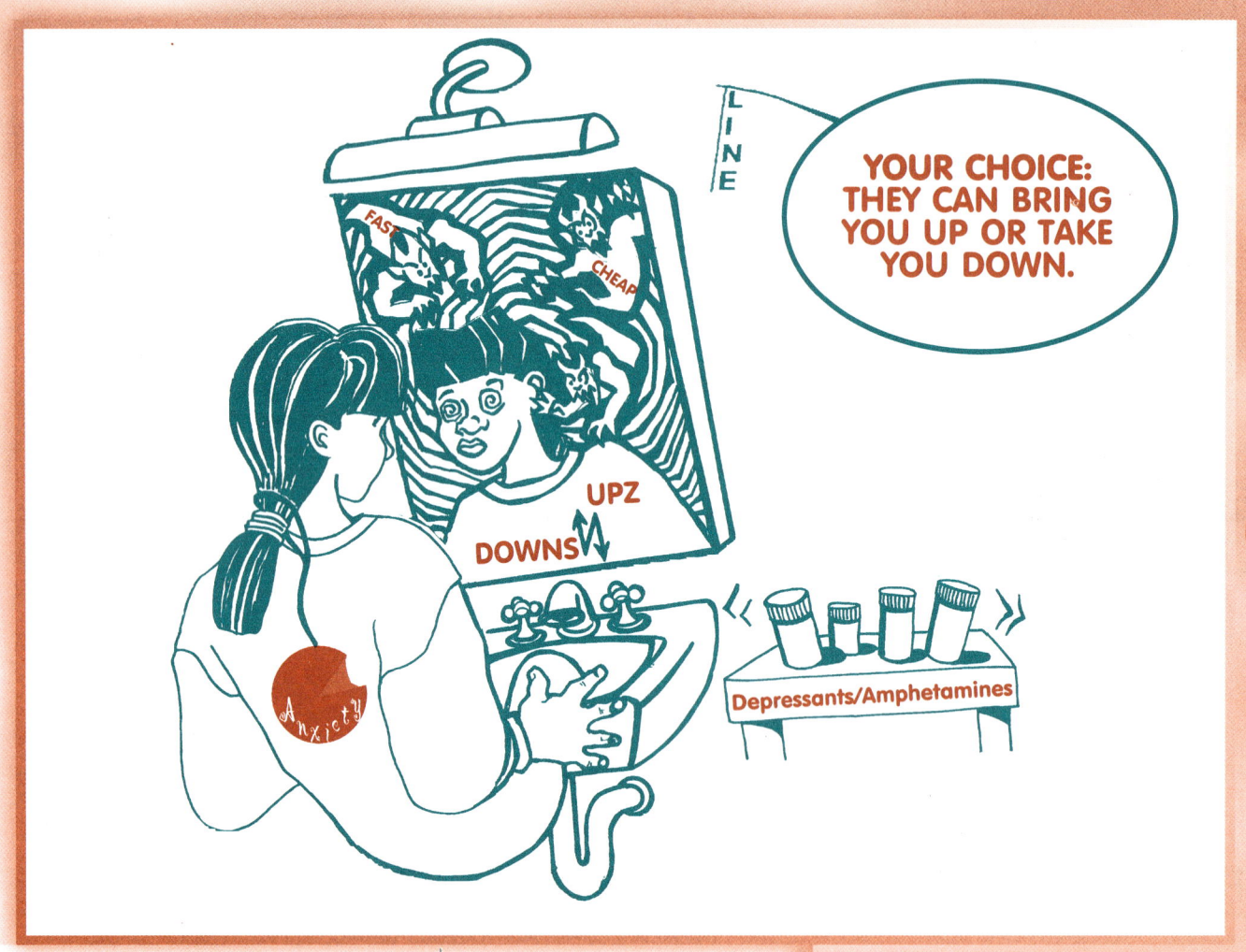

[Cartoon: A person with "Anxiety" on their shoulder looks into a mirror hanging over a sink. The mirror reflects a distressed face with "FAST" and "CHEAP" labels and "UPZ" / "DOWNS" arrows. On the counter sit bottles labeled "Depressants/Amphetamines." A speech bubble labeled LINE reads: "YOUR CHOICE: THEY CAN BRING YOU UP OR TAKE YOU DOWN."]

THINK ABOUT IT...

Use the cartoon above to answer the following questions:

HOOK — To what two drugs can abusers become dually addicted?

_____

LINE — What tempts teens to abuse these drugs?

_____

SINKER — What condition can result from dual addiction?

_____

Be Street Smart

View life positively.

Reduce stress by turning obstacles into opportunities!

For Advice And Information Call:

National Council on Alcoholism and Drug Dependence (NCADD)

1-800-NCA-Call
or
http://www.ncadd.org

AMPHETAMINES/DEPRESSANTS

CHECKUP

MATCHING

Column A	Column B
1. ___ amphetamines	a. drugs that "speed" a person up
2. ___ tranquilizers	b. illegal amphetamine-type drug
3. ___ barbiturates	c. drugs that calm a person down
4. ___ adrenaline	d. natural hormone made by body that prepares person for fight or flight
5. ___ ice	e. sleeping pills

FILL IN THE BLANKS

adrenaline   stress   blood
fatal   relax   sleep   slow   functions

Amphetamines are a group of drugs that "speed up" body_____. They cause the unnatural release of_____ into a person's body. Too much adrenaline puts great _____ on a person. Abusers run the risk of damaging _____ vessels. Depressants are a group of drugs that _____ down a person's brain and nervous system. Tranquilizers cause a person to _____. Barbiturates cause a person to_____. If these drugs are mixed with alcohol, it can be _____.

MULTIPLE CHOICE

1. **A drug that makes a person feel as if they have more energy**
   a. barbiturate
   b. tranquilizer
   c. amphetamine

2. **A drug that makes a person feel sleepy**
   a. barbiturate
   b. adrenaline
   c. amphetamine

3. **A natural hormone in the body that gives a person extra energy**
   a. amphetamine
   b. adrenaline
   c. barbiturate

4. **When people abuse uppers and downers at the same time, they may**
   a. have a dual addiction
   b. have bad breath
   c. fall asleep easily

5. **During an emergency, adrenaline in the bloodstream produces a sudden rush of energy that is sometimes described as a "fight or flight" response to danger. This means that people**
   a. can fly
   b. can pilot an airplane
   c. have extra strength to fight or get away from danger

TAKE A STAND

Dear Mrs. D.

IMPROVE YOUR REFUSAL SKILLS

Dear Mrs. D.:
Ever since Jr. High School, I've been nervous and up tight. I'm shy and don't feel comfortable talking to guys. I'm not sure what to say or how to act.

Laura, my best friend, offered me some pills to help me relax. I didn't take them, but I was tempted. She's so popular and all the guys seem to like her.

What can I do to fit in?

Signed,
Tired of being shy

Write how you would answer if you were Mrs. D.

Mrs. D. Answers:
_____
_____
_____
_____
_____
_____
_____
_____
_____

Show that you recognize the danger by completing the exercise below.

DANGER

All the kids think Courtney's mom is really cool. She wears the latest styles. She always has her hair fixed "right.". She goes to the "right" stores, to the "right" clubs, and is friends with the "right" people. Courtney's mom expects Courtney to be the same way.

Courtney knows that her mom isn't as confident as she seems. She is never certain that she looks right, or will say the right thing. She takes uppers before going out. She is "wired" when she gets home, and can't relax so she takes a tranquilizer before dinner. A sleeping pill makes sure she gets to sleep.

1. **Underline** a sentence that shows abusive behavior by Courtney's mom.

2. **Circle** a sentence that shows how Courtney's mom is putting her at risk for drug abuse.

3. Write a sentence that tells how Courtney can avoid worrying like her mom. _____
_____
_____

Write the coolest way to say, "No!"

1. **The Offer** "Hey Ted, you look down. Here, pop a bennie."

   You say _____
   _____

2. **The Dare** "Yo, Amy, you're so out of it. Try some ice. Dare to be cool."

   You say _____
   _____

BACK OFF

3. **The Threat** "If you don't get some sleep soon, you're going to be wasted for the game tomorrow. Take these to help you sleep."

   You say _____
   _____

4. **The Feel Good Approach** "Johnny, you look uptight. Here's some "crank" to help you chill."

   You say _____
   _____

AMPHETAMINES/DEPRESSANTS

Street Smarts

YOUR TURN

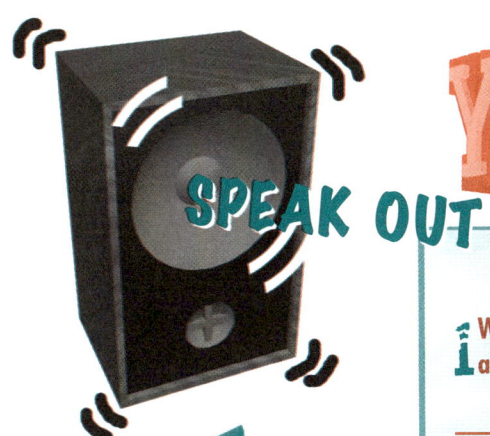

SPEAK OUT — LIGHTS, CAMERA, ACTION!

1. Why are some abusers who use amphetamines or depressants likely to become dually addicted?

2. What precautions can doctors take to make sure that their patients do not abuse tranquilizers and sleeping pills?

ASK A PARENT AN ADULT GUARDIAN

ASK: Do you think it is too easy to get tranquilizers? What other alternatives can help people deal with stress?

INTERACT

Setting: Your best friend Adam has confided to you that he has a dual addiction to sleeping pills and amphetamines. You have observed that his health has been getting worse. Adam wants help, but is afraid to go to his parents.

Situation: Adam needs professional help NOW!

Solution: Act out the scene between you and Adam. Make sure that you convince him that professional help is needed.

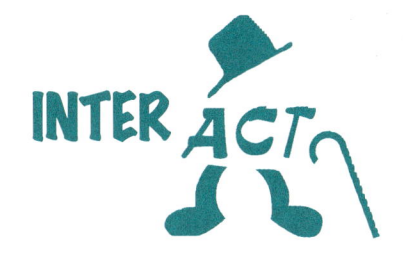

Teen Talk

1. You have noticed diet supplements at your local pharmacy that promise to reduce appetite and cause weight loss. How can you find out if they are safe? If they are not, how can you convince the pharmacy not to sell them?

2. What healthy recommendations could you make to an overweight friend who asked you for advice on losing weight?

INHALANTS
CHAPTER 11

THE BIG LIE

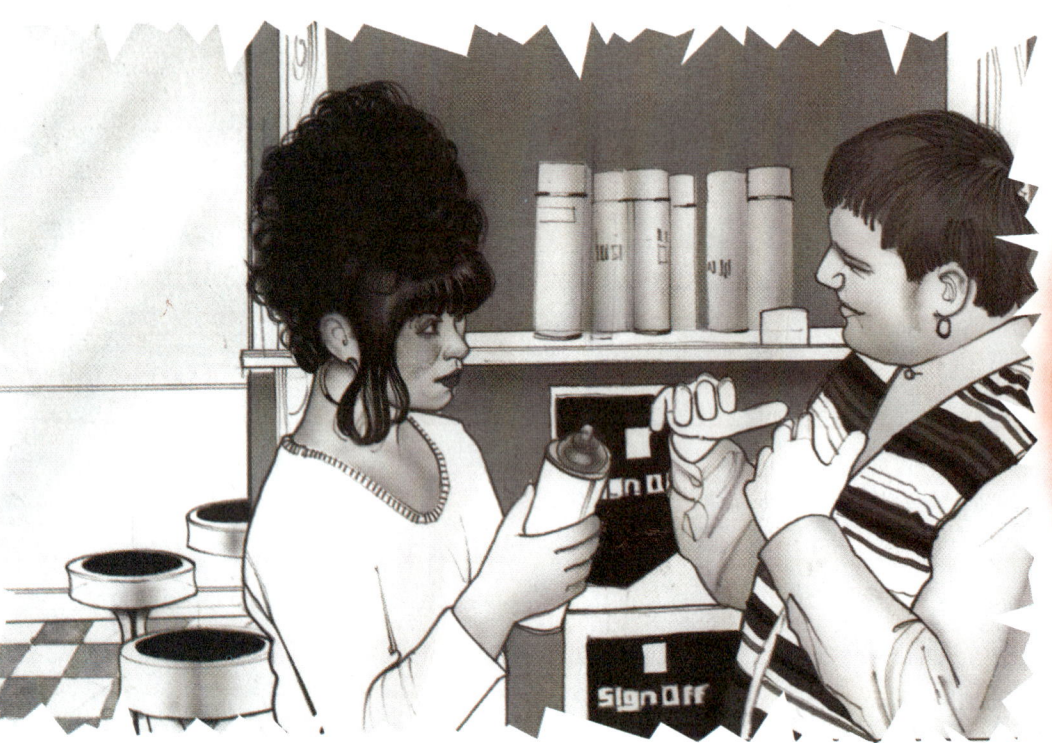

"BE HONEST. STOP LYING TO YOURSELF"

Tommy looked around the empty parking lot behind Mr. Rodriquez's bodega. A few cars were parked there, but not the one he was looking for. Tommy slumped in his seat. "I guess she didn't believe I'd come," he thought. "What's the point of going in now," he wondered. He didn't know any of the "No-Mores."

It never crossed his mind that his girlfriend, Debra, wouldn't come. She had always been supportive even when he lied or made up pitiful excuses to cover the fact that he was sniffing inhalants. Now, more than ever, he wanted her to hear him admit what he had been doing. He recalled the day that she had confronted him.

They were both working at the ice cream shop. The shop was empty and Tommy was loading supplies onto the storeroom shelf. In a few minutes the counter would be crowded with kids on their way home from school. He checked Debra's location. She was cleaning the counter. Tommy eyed the box of whipped cream containers on the floor and reached for a can....

"Tommy, T-O-M-M-Y! I need some help out here," Debra called. No answer. Debra finished serving the last customer and headed for the storeroom.

"Tommy, who are you trying to kid? We've been going out for three months now. And we work here together six days a week. Don't you think that I know what you're doing? I was wrong not to say something sooner, to have to hear it from our boss, Mr. James, that's just too much."

Tommy placed another box of whipped cream containers on the stack. Without looking at Debra he answered, "Deb, trust me. Don't listen to old man James. I didn't do it. He's filling your brain with lies. No one gets high on whipped cream. I am not doing whippets."

Disappointment showed on Debra's face. "Tommy, Mr. James saw you sniffing the air from the whipped cream cans. He probably wouldn't have known to watch you if the supplier hadn't called about all the 'returns' on the whipped cream containers. The supplier said that there was no way that so many cans of whipped cream could go flat."

Tommy could hear the sadness in Debra's voice. "Can't you just admit it? Don't blame Mr. James. And don't lie to me. Be honest. Stop lying to yourself. Don't you want to help yourself?" Then, almost in tears, she added, "I can't believe you would lie to me."

Tommy pretended he was fixing his shoelace. He kicked the whipped cream container he had been using under the shelf and avoided looking directly at Debra. "Deb, you're making a big deal out of nothing. Let's just forget it."

No More Pretense

"Tommy, how can we pretend nothing has happened? You are sniffing to get high every day and then lying about it. I like you too much to stay with you and pretend. It's not fair to either of us. You think inhaling is no big deal but you're wrong. Besides losing your job, and probably me, you're taking a chance with your life. And don't kid yourself that you can stop on your own. You need help: serious help."

There was a heavy silence between them. Tommy could not decide what to do. His stomach felt like it was tied up in knots. He thought that perhaps if he admitted it, Deb wouldn't break up with him. At least she didn't know the other things he was inhaling. She would think he was really crazy sniffing glue, paint, and deodorant. He had to admit that he felt some relief that she had found out. He knew that his sniffing was getting out of control.

Debra broke the silence. "I know what you're thinking. Your brother called me. We talked about you. He told me that he found rags and spray cans in your bedroom closet. I told him about the whipped cream containers here. We both agreed that if you decided to go for help, we would stick by you. We will. But ONLY if you go for help."

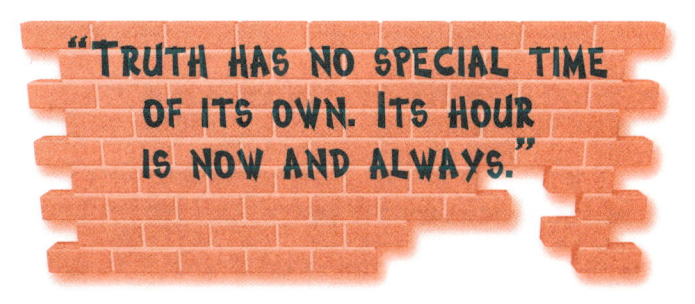

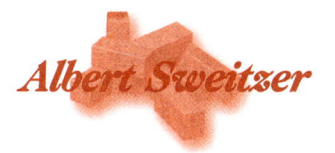

"TRUTH HAS NO SPECIAL TIME OF ITS OWN. ITS HOUR IS NOW AND ALWAYS."

Albert Sweitzer

TELL IT

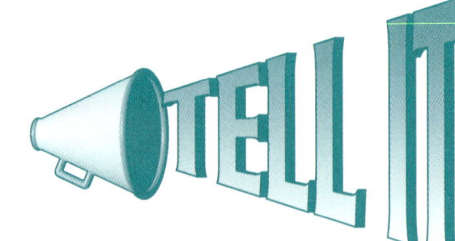

The Breath Of Life

Most of us take breathing for granted since it happens automatically. Oxygen is taken in when we inhale. It is rushed to our brain and all other body cells. Carbon dioxide waste is removed from all the cells and passed out when we exhale. The respiratory system is the wonderful life support system that gives us the oxygen we can't live without for more than a few minutes.

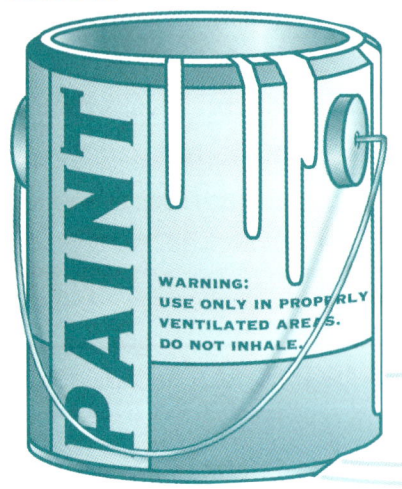

Inhalants are drugs that interfere with this life support system. As inhalants rush into the air passages, the toxic fumes enter directly into the blood and go instantly to the brain. In this way, they very quickly affect the body.

Special Warnings

Some common names for inhalants are solvents, nitrates, giggle gas, sniff, whippets and poppers. Some people accidently misuse these common household products. Petroleum-based products like gasoline, paint thinners, lighter fluid, degreasers, glues, adhesives, nail polish remover and household cleansers give off dangerous fumes. Direct inhalation of these products must be avoided. To prevent danger, make sure these products are used in well-ventilated areas only.

Aerosol cans that produce spray mists also pose a threat when used improperly. Inhalation of these mists can be extremely dangerous. Common household aerosol spray products include hair sprays, canned deodorants and spray paints. Because of danger of accidental inhalation, most of these products include special labels cautioning people about proper use. Aerosols, like petroleum products, must also be used in well-ventilated places only.

Don't Waste Your Breath

Some people purposely abuse inhalants. Often, they are too young to realize the serious dangers involved. Young teens, even elementary school students, sometimes inhale fumes from glue, paint, gasoline or other chemicals to get high. When inhaled, the chemical fumes from the products take the place of oxygen. As a result, the brain and other body parts do not receive the oxygen they need.

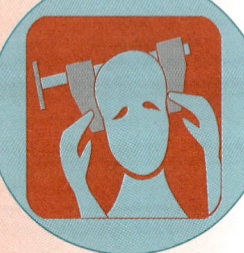

Inhalants can cause feelings of silliness or relaxation that last a short period of time. After these feelings pass, many abusers experience nausea, dizziness, nosebleeds, headaches, blurred vision, and even loss of coordination. Using large amounts of inhalants in a short period of time can cause violent behavior, suffocation or even death. Continued long-term use can result in weight loss, damage to the liver, kidney and heart, as well as permanent brain damage.

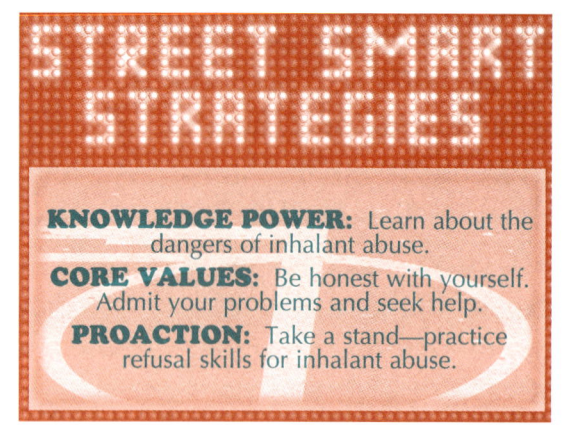

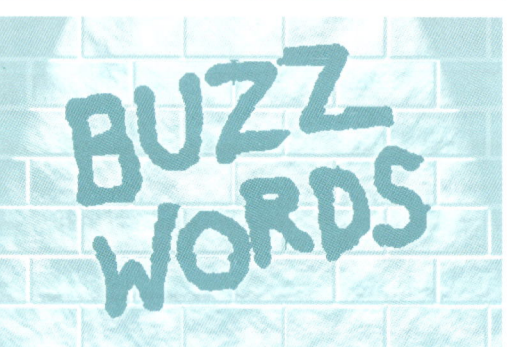

WARNING: USE ONLY IN PROPERLY VENTILATED AREAS. DO NOT INHALE.

STREET SMART STRATEGIES

KNOWLEDGE POWER: Learn about the dangers of inhalant abuse.
CORE VALUES: Be honest with yourself. Admit your problems and seek help.
PROACTION: Take a stand—practice refusal skills for inhalant abuse.

BUZZ WORDS

1. Breathing — taking in oxygen, pushing out carbon dioxide
2. Exhale — breathe out
3. Fumes — gases or vapors given off by chemicals
4. inhale — breathe in
5. Inhalant — substances with fumes inhaled for a special effect
6. Interfere — get in the way of something or someone
7. Nausea — feeling sick to your stomach
8. Suffocation — to die from a lack of oxygen
9. Toxic — poisonous
10. Ventilated — getting fresh air

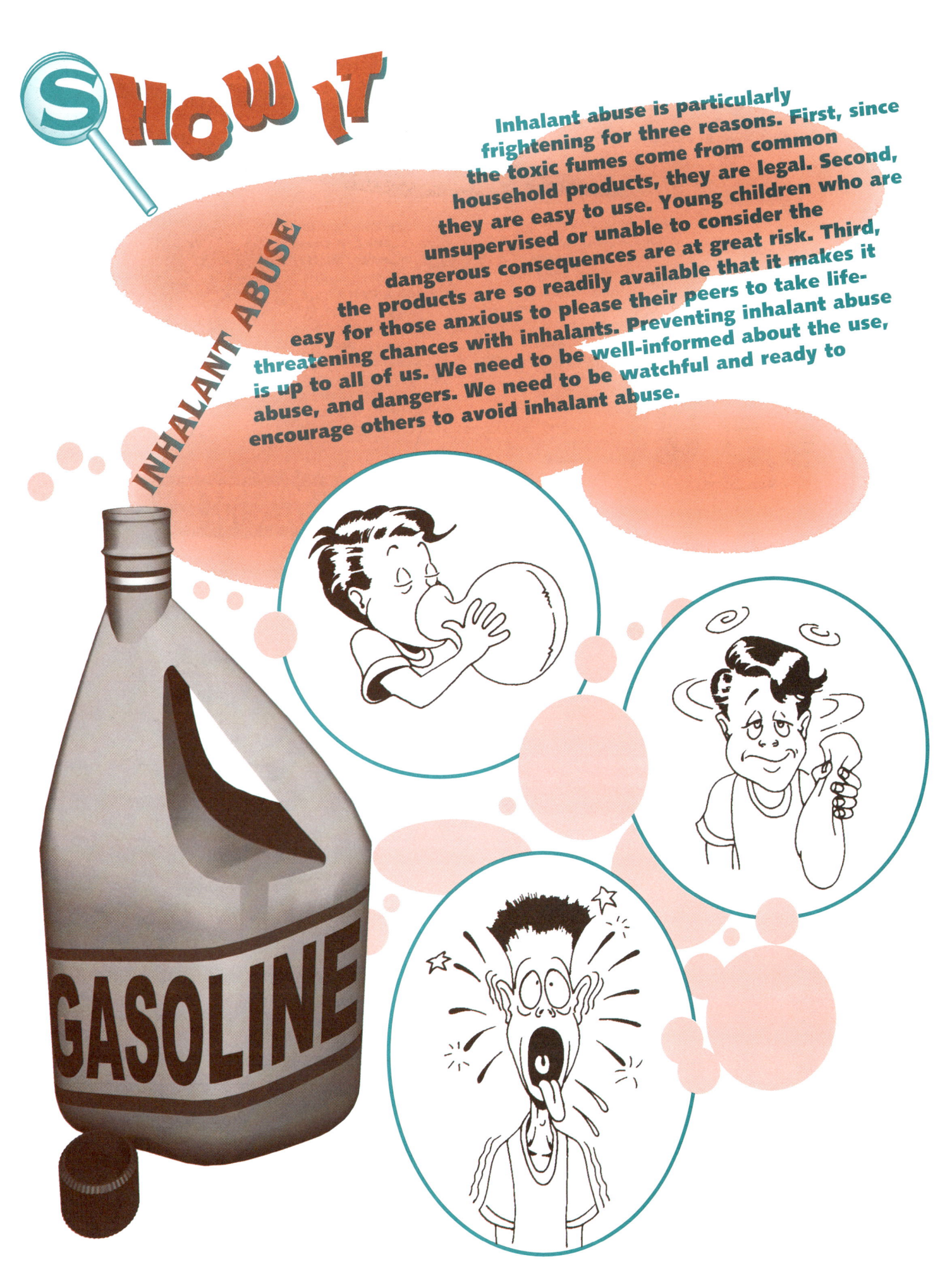

Show It

Inhalant Abuse

Inhalant abuse is particularly frightening for three reasons. First, since the toxic fumes come from common household products, they are legal. Second, they are easy to use. Young children who are unsupervised or unable to consider the dangerous consequences are at great risk. Third, the products are so readily available that it makes it easy for those anxious to please their peers to take life-threatening chances with inhalants. Preventing inhalant abuse is up to all of us. We need to be well-informed about the use, abuse, and dangers. We need to be watchful and ready to encourage others to avoid inhalant abuse.

Show It: Facts About Inhalants

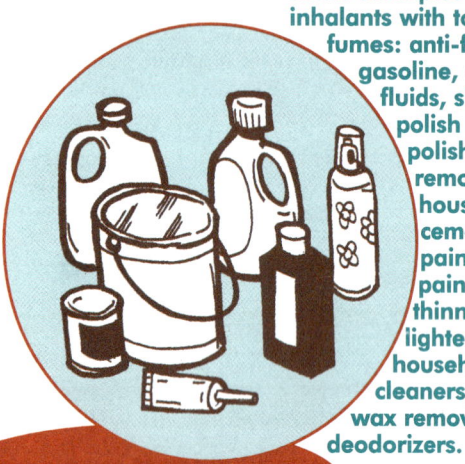

WHAT THEY ARE
Some examples of inhalants with toxic fumes: anti-freeze, gasoline, cleaning fluids, shoe polish and nail polish remover, household cement, paint and paint thinners, lighter fluid, household cleaners, floor wax removers, deodorizers.

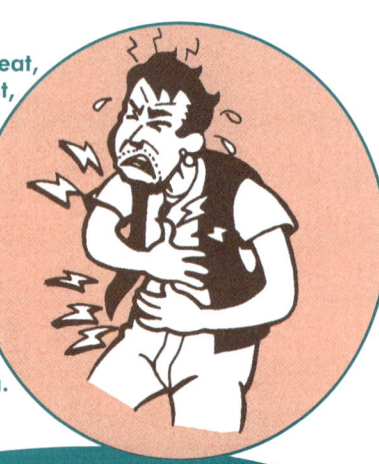

HOW THEY MAY AFFECT THE BODY
Increased heartbeat, pains in chest, muscles, joints; hangover, even amnesia; liver and kidney damage; respiratory damage; bone damage; blood cell damage; sleep disorders; nosebleeds; nausea; diarrhea.

WHAT THEY MAY CAUSE
Dizziness, a "rush," "drunk" feeling; weightlessness, silliness, slurred speech and poor coordination; sensitivity to light, enlarged pupils, double vision; ringing sound in ears; drowsiness, sleep; loss of appetite; violent behavior.

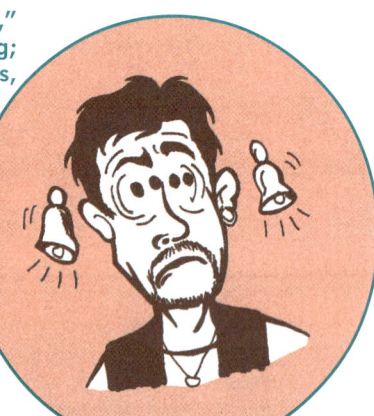

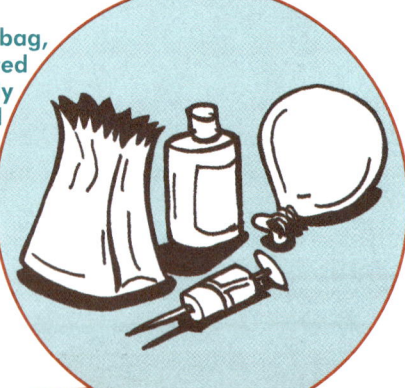

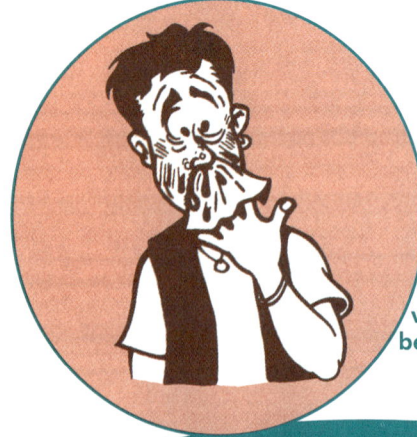

HOW THEY ARE USED
Inhaled from paper bag, balloon, or saturated material; inhaled directly from the container; mixed in alcoholic drinks and swallowed.; injected into veins; inhaling fumes in poorly ventilated area.

POSSIBLE SYMPTOMS OF ABUSE
Sniffer's rash," sores on nose and mouth; nosebleeds; strange or violent behavior.

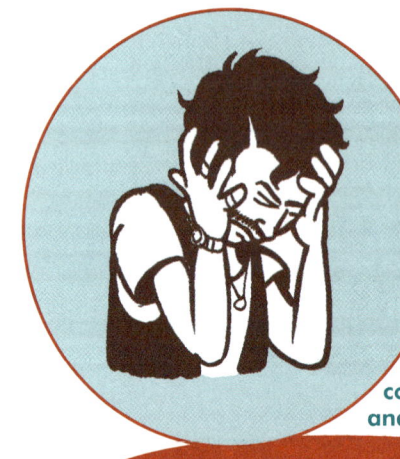

HOW THEY MAY AFFECT THE MIND
Nerve and brain damage; severe headaches; hallucinations, strange behavior. Disorientation, depression, seizures, coma, and death.

94   INHALANTS   Street Smarts

HOOK, LINE, AND SINKER

HOOK: The drugs that get people hooked. **LINE:** The lie that gets them to take the drugs. **SINKER:** The bad results of taking drugs.

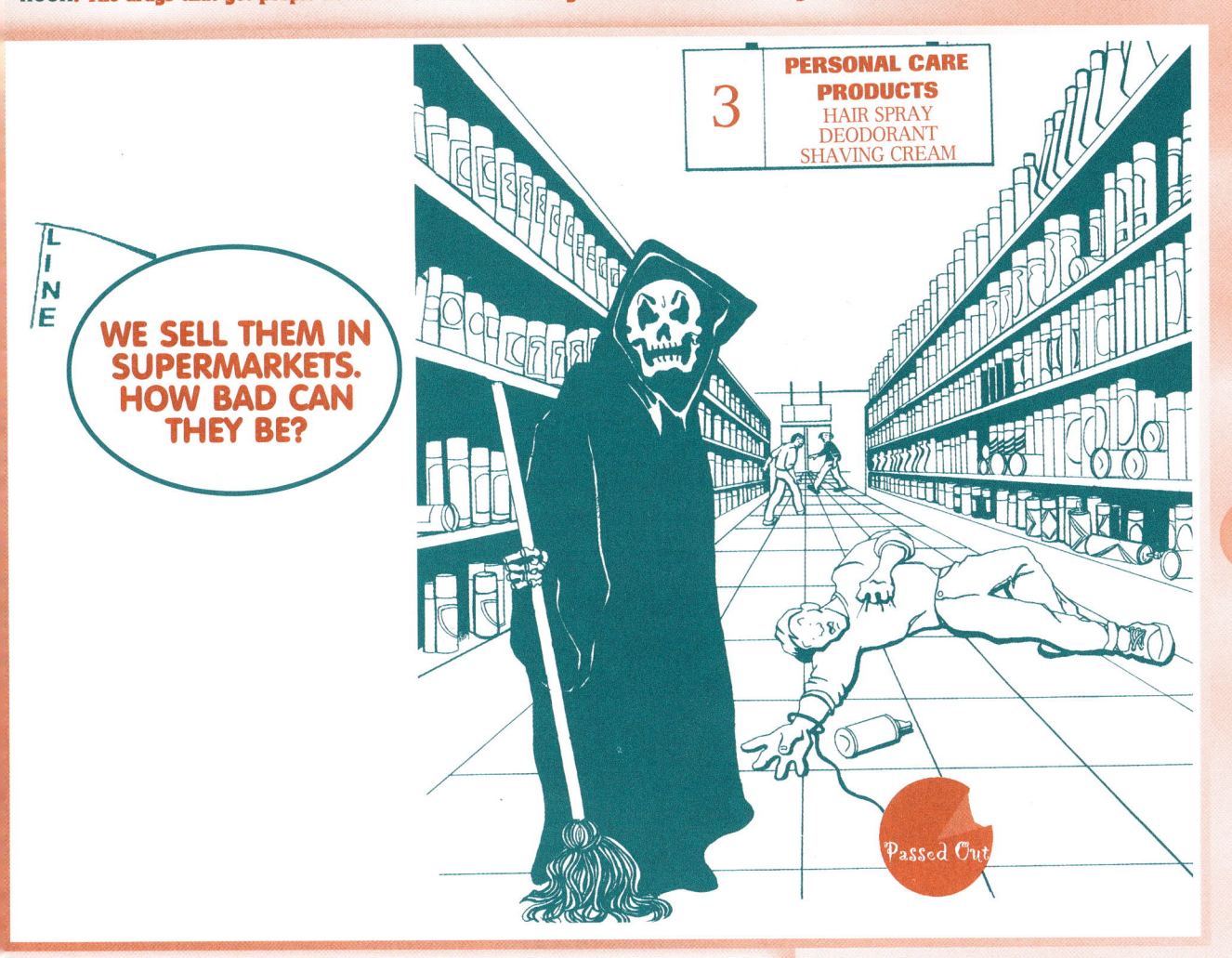

LINE

"WE SELL THEM IN SUPERMARKETS. HOW BAD CAN THEY BE?"

3 — PERSONAL CARE PRODUCTS
HAIR SPRAY
DEODORANT
SHAVING CREAM

Passed Out

THINK ABOUT IT...

Use the cartoon above to answer the following questions:

HOOK: List two personal care products that can be abused.

LINE: How can teens be deceived into thinking that abuse of personal care products is not dangerous?

SINKER: What effect did this inhalant have on the abuser?

Be Street Smart

Don't waste your breath!

Breathing even small amounts of inhalants can KILL!

For Advice And Information Call:

National Council on Alcoholism and Drug Dependence (NCADD)

1-800-NCA-Call
or
http://www.ncadd.org

THE PEOPLES PUBLISHING GROUP, 1-800-822-1080. COPYING PROHIBITED BY LAW.

CHECKUP

MATCHING

Column A | Column B
1. ___ suffocate | a. to breathe air in
2. ___ ventilate | b. to breathe air out
3. ___ inhale | c. drug inhaled for special effect
4. ___ inhalant | d. to give fresh air
5. ___ exhale | e. to keep from breathing

FILL IN THE BLANKS

**feel   brain   inhalants   organ
suffocation   silliness   sniff   dizziness**

Inhalant abusers _____ chemicals to change the way that they _____. The _____ quickly enter the blood and travel to the _____. Some immediate results are _____ and _____. Continued abuse may cause _____ damage or _____.

MULTIPLE CHOICE

1. **Which of these products can be used as an inhalant?**
   a. oven cleaner
   b. cleaning spray
   c. both a and b

2. **What is a well-ventilated area?**
   a. area with fresh air
   b. closed-off room
   c. large area without windows

3. **What side effects are possible?**
   a. headaches, dizziness, eye watering
   b. improved eyesight
   c. increased memory

4. **Repeated overexposure can cause**
   a. permanent brain damage
   b. nervous system damage
   c. both a & b

5. **What might result from intentionally inhaling the fumes?**
   a. death
   b. ventilation
   c. well-being

TAKE A STAND

Dear Mrs. D.

IMPROVE YOUR REFUSAL SKILLS

Dear Mrs. D.:
Me and my friends got a job at a restaurant busing tables. The money is good but it's hard work carrying all those trays. The thing is, I'm saving for a car and I want to keep this job. But my buddies, they don't care. Whenever they get a chance, they run in the back where the guy fixes desserts. They grab the whipped cream containers and get high off the gas. They act like total idiots and they try to get me to join them. What should I do?

Signed,
Like living

Write how you would answer if you were Mrs. D.

Mrs. D. Answers:
_____
_____
_____
_____
_____
_____
_____
_____
_____

Show that you recognize the danger by completing the exercise below.

Your best friend Ronnie collects model airplanes and model cars. He builds the models in his basement using airplane glue. While visiting Ronnie, you notice several brown bags scattered around the table. At first, you don't think much about it because Ronnie often keeps parts of models inside them.

You are called away from the basement to answer a phone call. When you return, you decide to "sneak up" on Ronnie as a trick. As you quietly come down the stairs, you see Ronnie with a brown bag over his nose and mouth. As Ronnie sees you, he holds up the bag and offers you a whiff.

1. <u>Underline</u> a sentence that shows Ronnie is abusing inhalants.

2. (Circle) a sentence that shows how Ronnie's behavior could put you at risk.

3. Write a sentence that tells what you should do. _____
_____

Write the "coolest" way to say, "No!"

1. **The Offer** "Jerry, I got a can of spray paint. No one's home. Let's sniff and get high."

   You say _____
   _____

2. **The Dare** "The manager is not looking. I dare you to get high from that canister in the whipped cream case."

   You say _____
   _____

3. **The Threat** "What do you mean you don't want to. If you don't, I'll tell about the last time you did it."

   You say _____
   _____

4. **The Feel Good Approach** "No need to feel down, I have something in this bag that will perk you up. Don't worry it's safer and it's not drugs."

   You say _____
   _____

BACK OFF

THE PEOPLES PUBLISHING GROUP, 1-800-822-1080. COPYING PROHIBITED BY LAW.

YOUR TURN

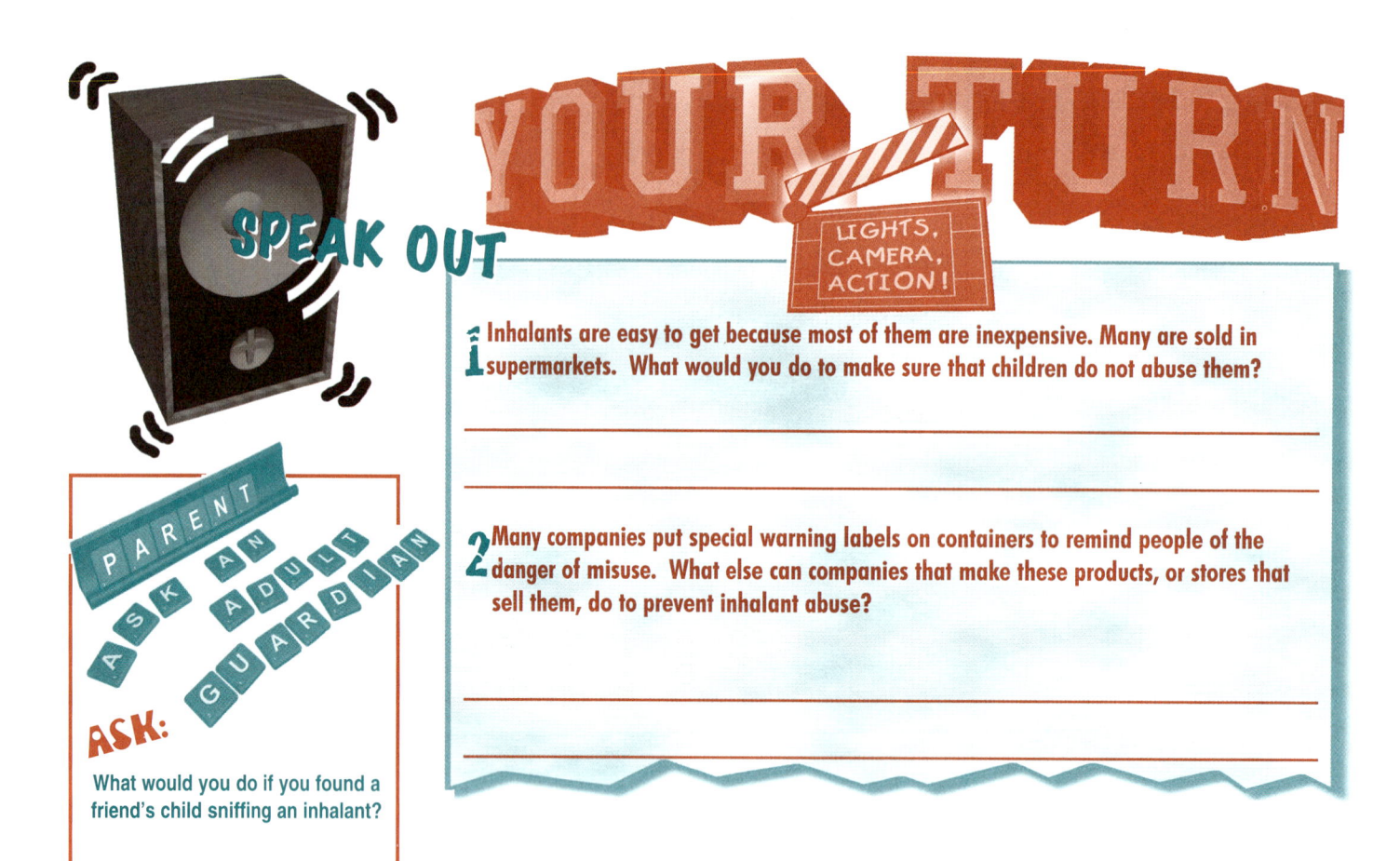

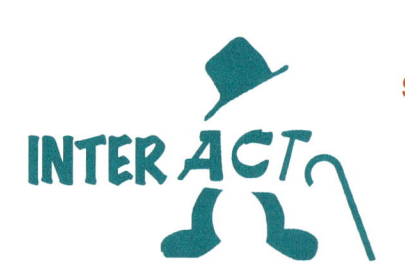

SPEAK OUT

1. Inhalants are easy to get because most of them are inexpensive. Many are sold in supermarkets. What would you do to make sure that children do not abuse them?
   _____
   _____

2. Many companies put special warning labels on containers to remind people of the danger of misuse. What else can companies that make these products, or stores that sell them, do to prevent inhalant abuse?
   _____
   _____

ASK A PARENT AN ADULT GUARDIAN

ASK: What would you do if you found a friend's child sniffing an inhalant?

INTERACT

Setting: You are part of the drug-free teen group sent to talk to fifth and sixth-grade students.

Situation: After the group presentation, teachers give junior high students a chance to talk privately with your group. You find out that there is a lot of inhalant abuse, mostly gasoline and sprays.

Solution: What is your responsibility to the students? your group? the school? Act out: (1) What you will say to the students? (2) What you will say to the teachers?

Teen Talk

1. What can communities do to help educate and prevent inhalant abuse?
   _____
   _____
   _____

2. The girl who has the locker next to you at school keeps inhalants in the bottom of her locker. Between classes, when she thinks no one is looking, she sniffs. What do you do or say? To whom?
   _____
   _____
   _____

CHAPTER 12

OVER-THE-COUNTER/PRESCRIPTION DRUGS

WEIGH IN OR WAY OUT

Derrick spotted Darrell with someone new and walked over. "I know you. You're from Central High. You're on the wrestling team, aren't you?" Derrick asked.

Ron looked up in surprise. He hadn't expected anyone to recognize him here. And he certainly wasn't planning to get into it with anyone on his first night. He answered, "Nope, I'm not on any wrestling team."

Nowhere To Hide

"Central High School hung our team out to dry," Derrick continued. "And I'm sure I saw you pin one of our best guys. You were on that team. I know you were. So, why are you hiding it?"

Ron could not hide his annoyance. "What do you know? Are you trying to say I'm crazy?"

"Hey, cool it. Let's keep this on the down-low. Look man, nobody's trying to hassle you or make you say nothing," Darrel said calmly. "We're just

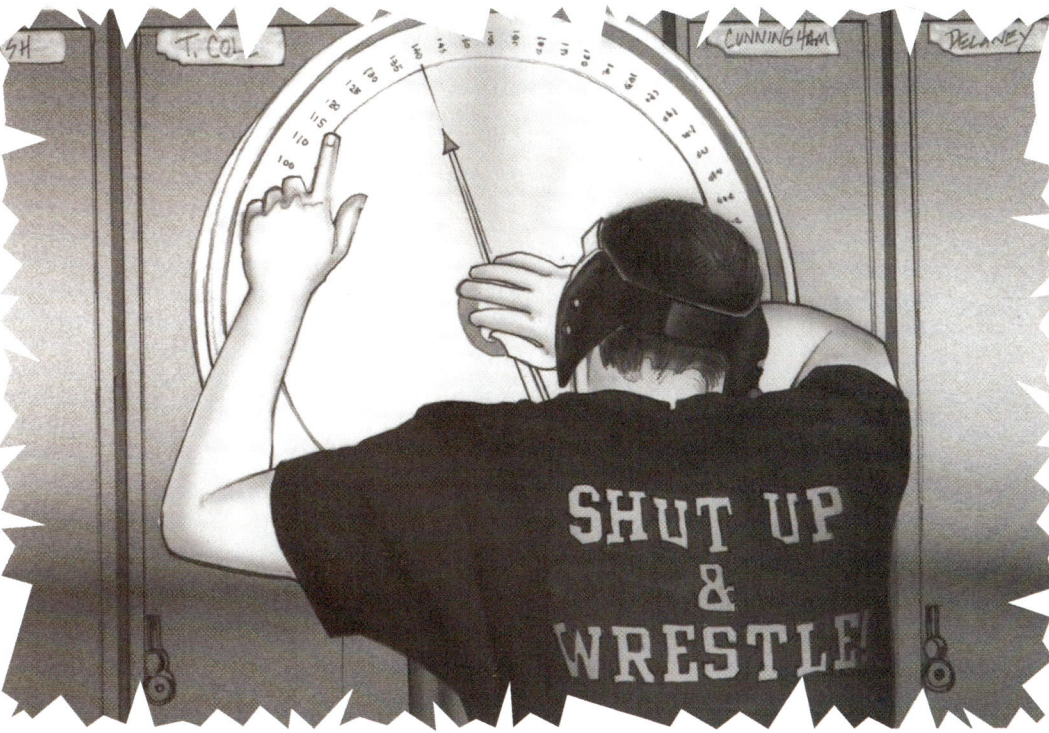

"I was looking for an answer.... An easy way, so I could eat and keep the weight down."

interested. Isn't that right, Derrick?"

Derrick turned to walk away. Ron stepped forward, stuck his hand in Derrick's direction and said, "The name's Ron, Ron Jerrard. Sorry. I don't like people poking around in my business. Since my last match, it seems like everyone's trying to get into my personal life. I didn't mean to be rude, I just never expected anyone to recognize me here."

"You don't look like a druggie and I bet the courts didn't send you here either," Derrick responded. What's the deal? Why are you here?

Pinned By A Habit

Ron was silent for a while before he answered. "In wrestling you lose if you get pinned, right? Well, I got pinned big time, only not the way you think. I had to wrestle at 120 pounds, that's my limit. Any higher and I go into the next weight class. Those guys are much bigger than me. There's no way I could take them, so I constantly had to diet to keep my weight down. Only, I was hungry all the time; all I could think of was food."

"As the wrestling matches got closer, I got scared. I was afraid I wouldn't make the team. I started taking diet pills, but I was still hungry all the time. Then I came up with an easy way to eat and keep my weight down. I started taking laxatives and I'd make myself vomit. I also kept taking the diet pills as added insurance."

"Everything seemed to be working fine. Well, I was wrong: I almost killed myself. I was eating like a horse and then getting rid of it. I didn't realize I was messing up my system."

"My last wrestling match came and I weighed in fine. I was all set to go. Then my heart started racing like crazy, I passed out and had to be taken to the emergency room. I realize now that I had pinned myself with my bad habits!"

"That was a couple of months ago. Since then, I've been with a bunch of girls in the Eating Disorder Clinic at North Forks Hospital. For a while, I wondered if I was the only male bulimic in the world. But I bet there are enough other bulimic wrestlers to make a team. Bulimia is addictive and I've got to be really careful."

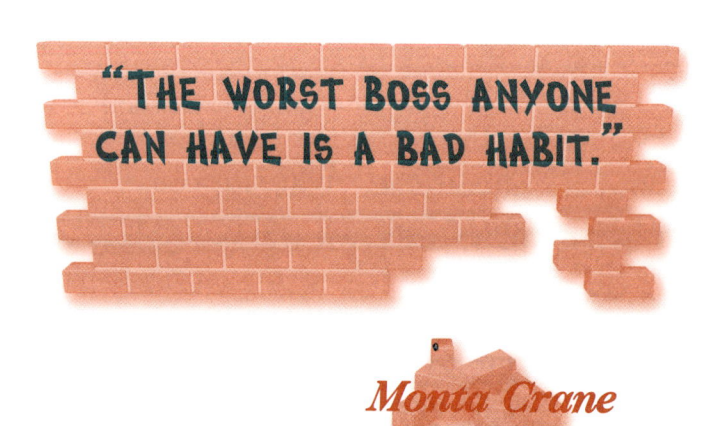

"THE WORST BOSS ANYONE CAN HAVE IS A BAD HABIT."

Monta Crane

TELL IT

Rx For Health

The human body is very complex. Billions of cells work together, doing their own special job In order for us to survive. Food, oxygen, water, and waste must be continually moved. Cells that break down must be replaced. Harmful disease cells must be fought off and destroyed so that we don't get sick. While all this is going on, we must be able to respond to the outside world. Our thoughts, emotions, even our beliefs help us to do this. Our brain acts like the master computer in our body and coordinates all actions and thoughts.

The defense system that keeps us healthy is called the immune system. When disease cells enter or invade our body, the immune system goes into action to fight and destroy the invaders. Our behaviors can help our immune systems stay healthy. Eating balanced meals, drinking plenty of water, exercising, getting enough sleep, and having a positive attitude all contribute to keeping our immune systems in good working condition.

Rx Prescription

codeine - .40%

directions: take no more than one capsule every 24 hours as needed for pain relief.

When Invaders Win

Usually our immune system does a good job of helping us stay fit. If the invaders (disease germs) take control, we feel sick and may need medical help. After an examination, your doctor may write a prescription for a medicine to help your body fight the disease.

Over-The-Counter Medicines

For minor problems, extra sleep and liquids may be all that are needed. Sometimes, doctors may suggest a product from the pharmacy called Over-the-Counter (OTC) medicine. Although a prescription from a doctor is not needed for an OTC, it is wise to talk to your doctor or pharmacist before deciding to use one. Allergies, special diets, or medical conditions might make an OTC dangerous for you. If it is decided that an OTC might be helpful, be certain to follow all directions carefully. Pregnant or nursing mothers should NEVER take any medicine — even over-the-counter — without a doctor's advice.

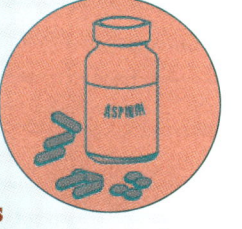

STREET SMART STRATEGIES

KNOWLEDGE POWER: Learn about the dangers of prescription and non-prescription drug abuse.

CORE VALUES: Eat well, sleep well, and exercise. Develop good health habits.

PROACTION: Take a stand—practice refusal skills for improper use of prescription and non-prescription drugs.

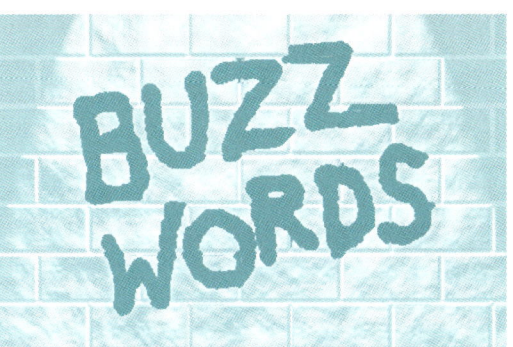

BUZZ WORDS

1. **Allergies** — body's negative reaction to a substance
2. **Bulimia** — an eating disorder that involves binging, vomiting and/or laxatives
3. **Coordinate** — work together
4. **Drug reactions** — the body's response to a drug
5. **Expiration date** — when the medicine should no longer be used
6. **Hypochondriac** — someone who imagines illness and may cause themselves to become sick
7. **Immune system** — the body's defense system that helps fight invading germs
8. **Invade** — to attack
9. **Medical history** — a record of medical illnesses and conditions that you have or once had
10. **OTC** — over-the-counter medicines
11. **Pharmacist** — trained professional who fills prescriptions
12. **Physician's Desk Reference (PDR)** — reference book that describes medical products and possible reactions
13. **Prescription** — note from a medical doctor for a particular medicine
14. **Symptoms** — signs that your body gives when your system is out of balance

Show It

Working with the Doctor

Before you see a doctor, you should prepare for the visit. Be aware of your symptoms. Plan to tell the doctor what you have been feeling and for how long. If this is a first visit, be sure to tell the doctor about your medical history and about any allergies or drug reactions you may have had. Ask the doctor if there are any alternatives besides drugs for handling the problem.

If the doctor feels you need medicine to help, he/she will give you a prescription. Prescription drugs are usually more powerful than OTC's. Be sure you understand how and when to take the medicine. Be aware of any changes you will need to make in your daily routine. For example, some drugs should be taken with meals. With others, you should avoid sunlight. Never mix prescription drugs with OTC's without a doctor's knowledge and approval.

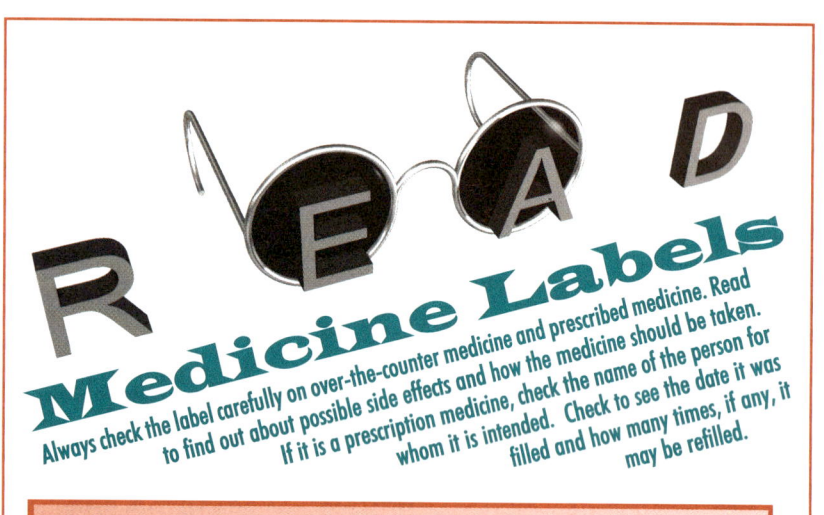

- Always let the doctor know if you are pregnant or nursing.
- If you break out in a rash or have any other bad reaction to a drug, call your doctor immediately!
- Always keep medicines away from children.
- Follow directions exactly.
- Never share medicines.
- Check the expiration date.

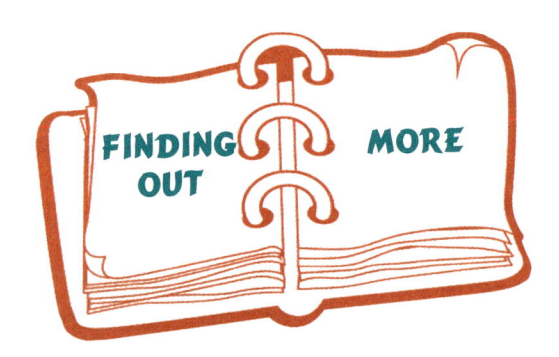

READ Medicine Labels

Always check the label carefully on over-the-counter medicine and prescribed medicine. Read to find out about possible side effects and how the medicine should be taken. If it is a prescription medicine, check the name of the person for whom it is intended. Check to see the date it was filled and how many times, if any, it may be refilled.

Rx LINCOLN PHARMACY
80 Lincoln Place
PHONE: 202-8768   #341334

JOHN JAY   DATE: 10/8/99

TAKE 1 TABLET, THREE TIMES A DAY. TAKE WITH MEALS.

WARNING: For adult use only. Do not give to children under 12 years. Do not exceed recommended dosage. Do not use for more than three days. If symptoms persist, consult a physician.

May cause dizziness. Do not drive or operate machinery.

Keep out of reach of children.

Store at room temperature.

RESPIRON COUGH SUPPRESSANT   NUMBER OF REFILLS: 0

Finding Out More

To learn more about a particular drug that a doctor has prescribed, ask your pharmacist to let you see the **Physicians Desk Reference** (PDR) or visit your library and read it. The PDR will describe the drug, along with any possible side affects.

Show It

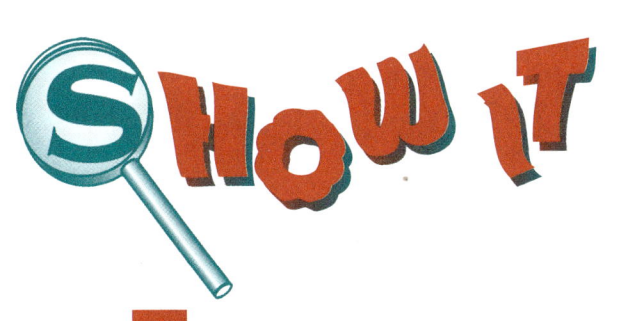

Work with your body to stay healthy. Healthy habits keep your immune system in good working order. If you should get sick, be responsible: discuss your symptoms with a parent or guardian. If symptoms persist, see a doctor.

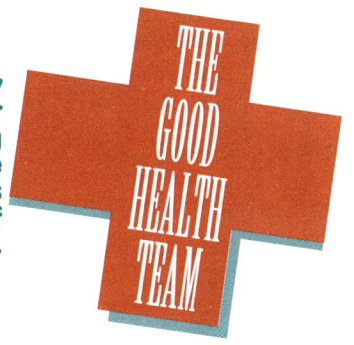

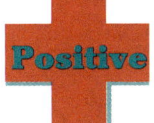

THE GOOD HEALTH TEAM

Positive Responses When You Feel Ill

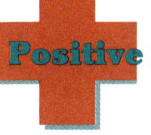

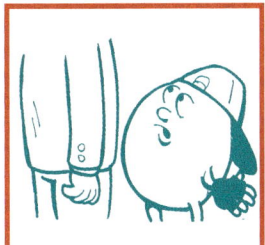

Talk to your parent/guardian about a doctor's visit.

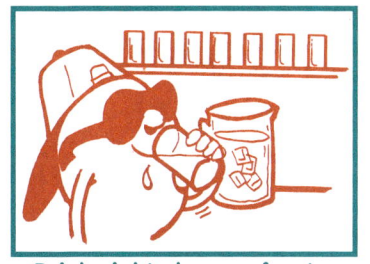

If you need medicine, do the following:

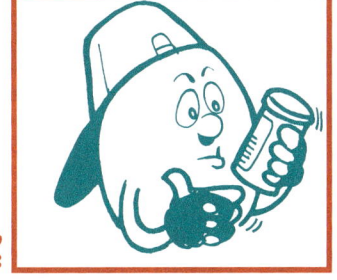

Read and follow directions.

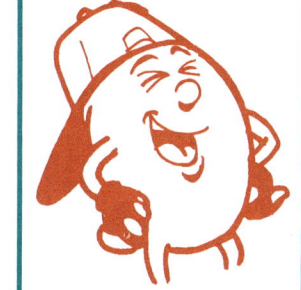

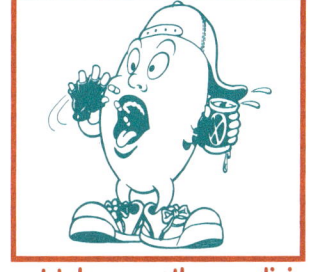

Do not take any other medicines or drugs.

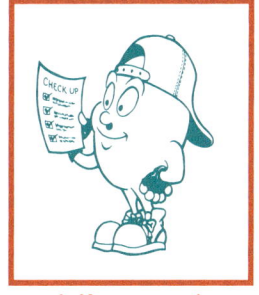

Ask if you need to return for a check-up.

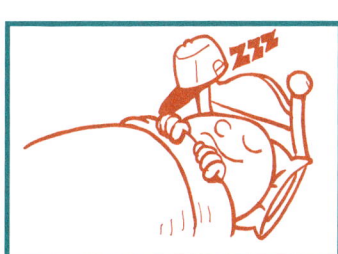

Follow your doctor's advice for care.

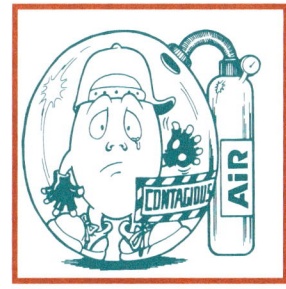

Ask if you are contagious, if so do not visit others.

Positive Habits To Stay Healthy

Drink eight glasses of water daily.

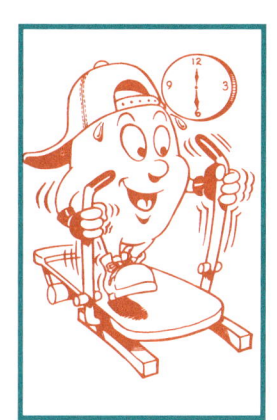

Exercise at least 30 minutes daily.

Maintain a healthful, positive attitude.

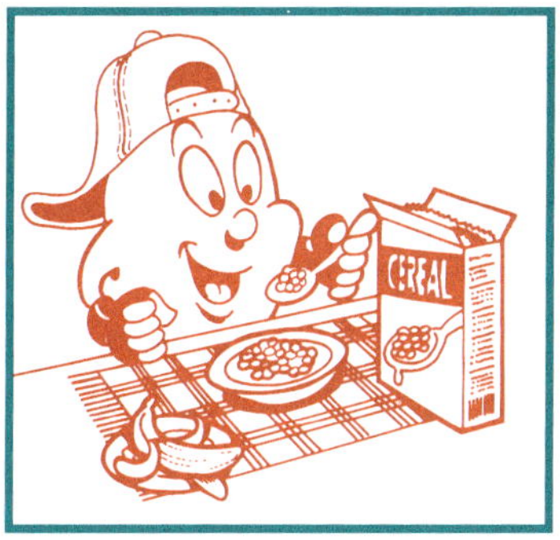

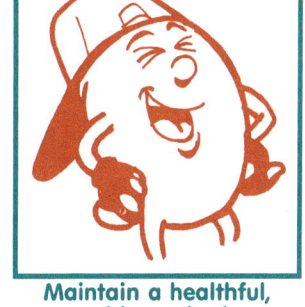

Eat a balanced diet.

Sleep 8 hours each night.

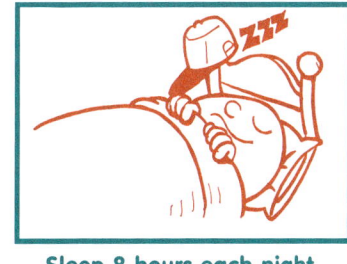

Develop relaxation skills.

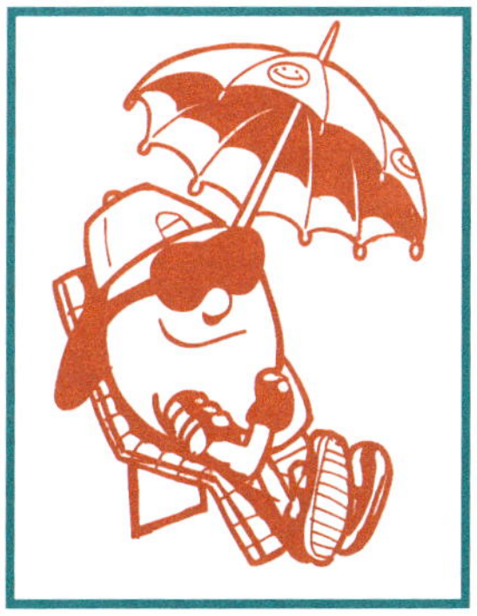

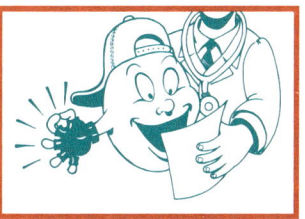

THE PEOPLES PUBLISHING GROUP, 1-800-822-1080. COPYING PROHIBITED BY LAW.

HOOK, LINE, AND SINKER

HOOK: The drugs that get people hooked. **LINE:** The lie that gets them to take the drugs. **SINKER:** The bad results of taking drugs.

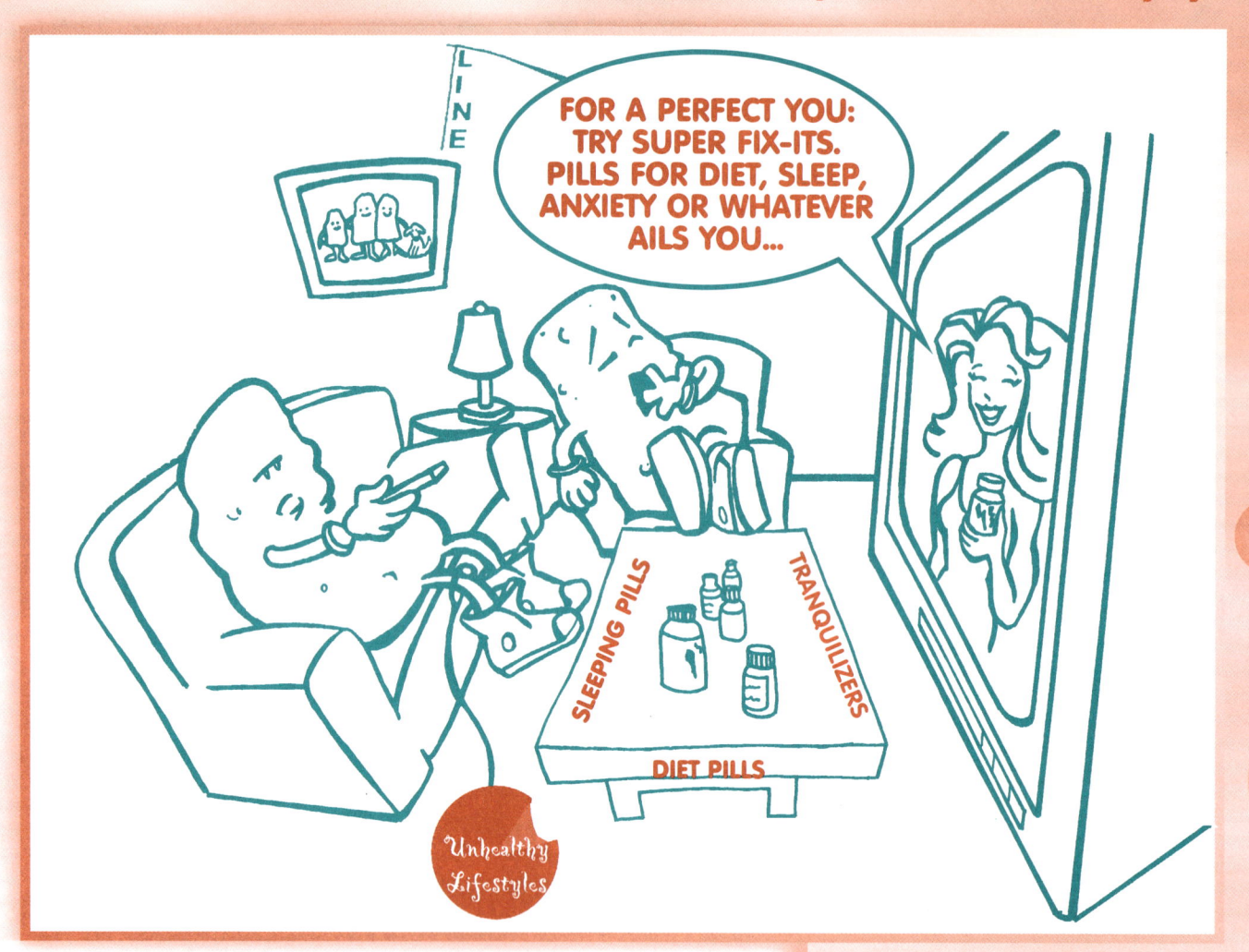

> LINE
>
> FOR A PERFECT YOU: TRY SUPER FIX-ITS. PILLS FOR DIET, SLEEP, ANXIETY OR WHATEVER AILS YOU...
>
> SLEEPING PILLS — TRANQUILIZERS — DIET PILLS
>
> *Unhealthy Lifestyles*

THINK ABOUT IT...

Use the cartoon above to answer the following questions:

HOOK — What did the couch potatoes buy to solve their problems?
_____
_____

LINE — How does the TV commercial try to influence the couch potatoes?
_____
_____

SINKER — What may result from relying on pills to solve all of life's problems?
_____
_____

Be Street Smart

There are no short cuts to good health.

Eat nutritious foods.
Get plenty of sleep.
Work out.
Educate yourself for good health.

For Advice And Information Call:

National Council on Alcoholism and Drug Dependence (NCADD)

1-800-NCA-Call
or
http://www.ncadd.org

PRESCRIPTION/OVER-THE-COUNTER MEDICATIONS — Street Smarts

CHECKUP

MATCHING

Column A	Column B
1. ___ OTC	a. signs
2. ___ prescription	b. Physician's Desk Reference
3. ___ side effect	c. bad reaction to a medicine
4. ___ PDR	d. Over-the-Counter medicine
5. ___ symptoms	e. doctor's note for medicine

FILL IN THE BLANKS

sleep   body   parent   doctor   directions   water   exercising   immune

The human _____ is complex. It has its own way of fighting off disease. The "first line of defense" of the body is called the _____ system. To help keep the immune system healthy, drink eight glasses of _____ every day. It is also important to eat balanced meals, get plenty of _____ each night, and keep your body in shape by _____. If you do get sick, talk to your _____ or guardian to help you decide if you need to see a doctor. If you need to take medicine, read the _____ carefully. Never share a prescription drug with anyone. If you have a bad reaction call your _____ immediately.

MULTIPLE CHOICE

1. **A medicine sold in pharmacies without a prescription is called:**
   a. immune
   b. complex
   c. over-the-counter

2. **A doctor's note telling the pharmacist what medicine is needed is called:**
   a. over-the-counter
   b. prescription
   c. PDR

3. **The system in our body that fights disease is the**
   a. immune system
   b. reproductive system
   c. respiratory system

4. **About how many glasses of water should you drink daily?**
   a. two
   b. fifteen
   c. eight

5. **Which of the following is bad for your health:**
   a. Seeing a doctor when you are feeling ill.
   b. Taking OTC medicines when you are pregnant.
   c. Sleeping eight hours a night

TAKE A STAND

Dear Mrs. D.

IMPROVE YOUR REFUSAL SKILLS

Dear Mrs. D.:
I'm concerned about my sister. Ever since she came home from college, she has been taking medicine for every little thing. The least problem, and she pops a pill. I looked at the bottles. Nothing is illegal. It's just that she thinks she's always sick and that one pill or another will make things better.

In school we learned that people who always think they are sick are "hypochondriacs". That's kind of a big word. It sounds scary. How do you help a hypochondriac?

Signed,
Living with a hypochondriac

Write how you would answer if you were Mrs. D.

Mrs. D. Answers:
_____
_____
_____
_____
_____
_____
_____
_____
_____

Show that you recognize the danger by completing the exercise below.

Patty was very excited to have been picked for the kick-line at school. That meant she would be performing with the kick-line team at all the football games.

She was anxious to be accepted by the team. Uniforms would be passed out in three weeks. Everyone had been bugging her to lose weight. Patty wanted to please them, but she also liked to eat.

One of the girls mentioned that she had to lose weight last year. She offered to give Patty some of her diet pills so she could take the weight off fast.

1. <u>Underline</u> a sentence that shows why Patty is at risk of drug abuse.

2. (Circle) a sentence that shows who is tempting her.

3. How can Patty healthfully take care of this situation? _____
_____
_____

Write the "coolest" way to say, "No!"

1. **The Offer** "Hey, Jack, your cough sounds bad. I've got some prescription cough syrup. I'll give you some."

   You say _____
   _____

2. **The Dare** "Ann, are you too chicken to try these diet pills?"

   You say _____
   _____

   BACK OFF

3. **The Threat** "Ronnie, if you don't lose 10 pounds before the Homecoming Dance, you can forget about going with me."

   You say _____
   _____

4. **The Feel Good Approach** "Sally, I have just what you need to make you feel better: here is something for your headache; this one is for your stuffy nose; and this one will help that upset stomach."

   You say _____
   _____

YOUR TURN

SPEAK OUT

1. What do you think is the best way for a doctor to handle a "hypochondriac" who is always asking for medication?

_____

_____

2. In what ways do advertisers in magazines and on TV commercials encourage "pill popping"?

_____

_____

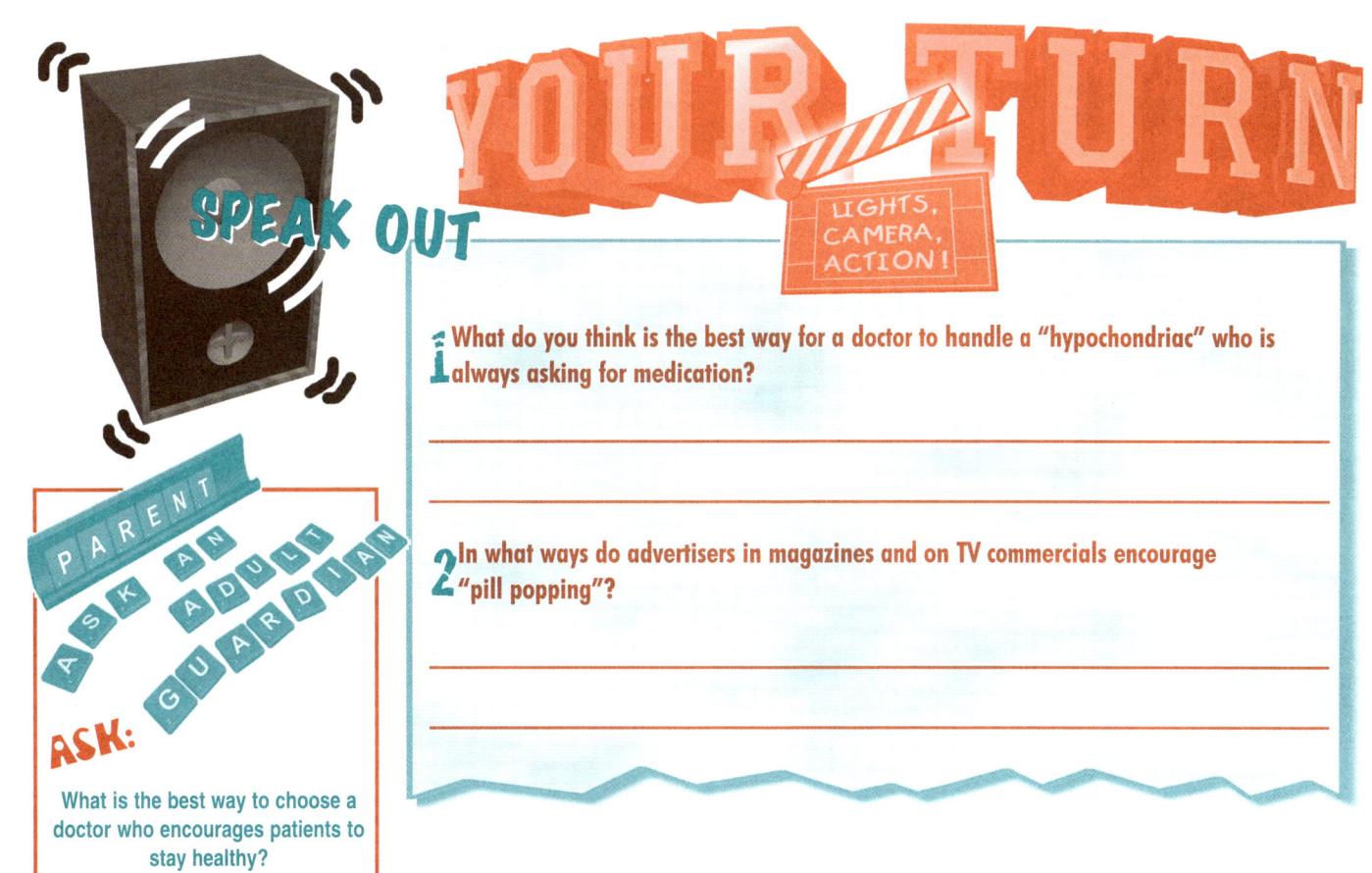

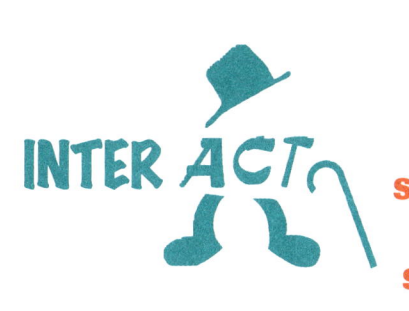

ASK A PARENT AN ADULT GUARDIAN

ASK: What is the best way to choose a doctor who encourages patients to stay healthy?

INTERACT

Setting: You are a member of the Healthy Life Styles Club at your school. As a part of Drug Awareness Week, you have been asked to plan an advertising campaign to encourage staff and students to develop positive health behaviors. You want to make sure that everyone understands that both legal and illegal drugs can be abused.

Situation: Meet with committee members and plan an advertising campaign. Stress positive behaviors and attitudes.

Solution: Act out the planning meeting with your committee. How will you get the message across?

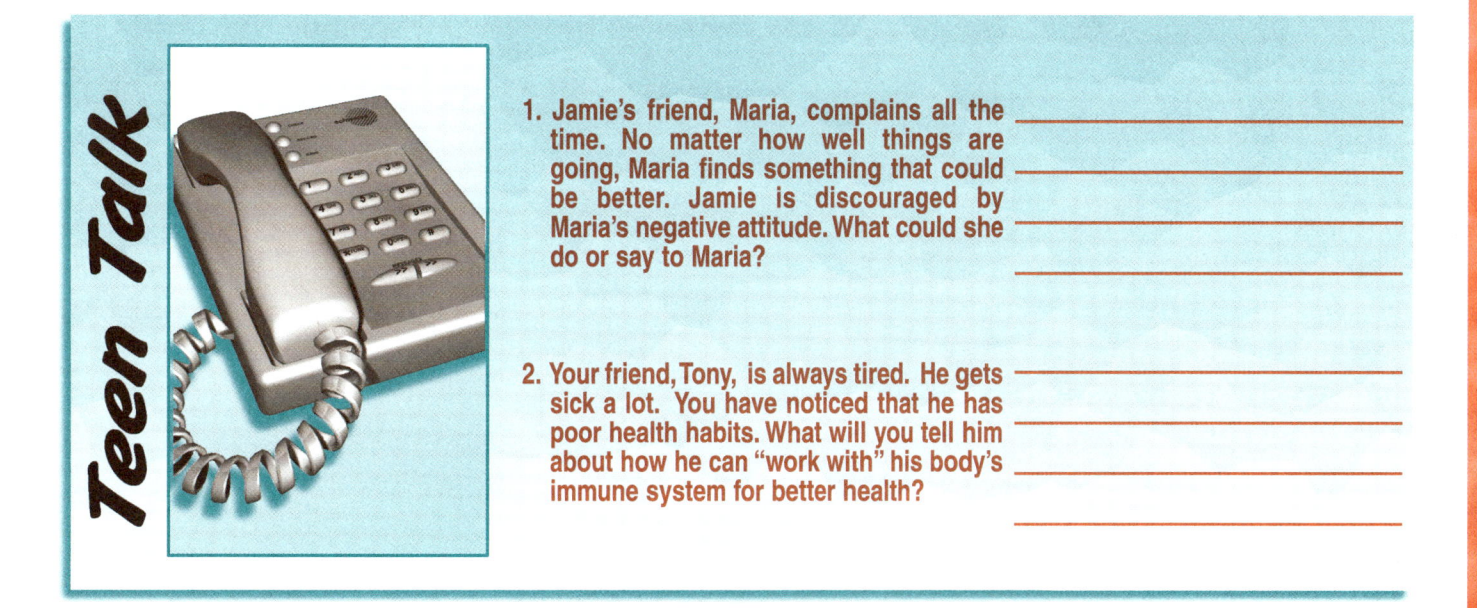

Teen Talk

1. Jamie's friend, Maria, complains all the time. No matter how well things are going, Maria finds something that could be better. Jamie is discouraged by Maria's negative attitude. What could she do or say to Maria?

2. Your friend, Tony, is always tired. He gets sick a lot. You have noticed that he has poor health habits. What will you tell him about how he can "work with" his body's immune system for better health?

HALLUCINOGENS
CHAPTER 13

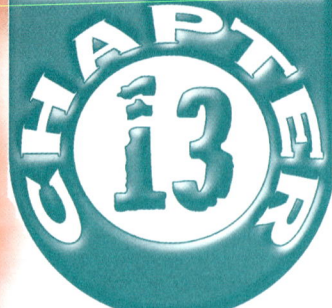

PCP SURPRISE

"I still can't believe it," Charles said, shaking his head. The photograph of Angela's swollen face on the front page of the newspaper was more than he could handle. He couldn't bring himself to read the words on the page.

"That's easy for you to say," Sharon fired back. "You were too 'dusted' to know what was really happening. Now that you've seen the paper, do you remember anything that happened that night?"

Party Madness

A sad look came over Charles' face, but he responded, "The truth is, I don't remember most of it. Only some parts, before and after," he said feebly.

"It started out as a great party. I was happy that all my friends were there. Of course, it was a little wild since Angela's parents were away for the weekend. I had gotten some pot, and as a special surprise, had some joints dipped in PCP. I waited until everyone was feeling good, then passed them out to anyone who wanted to get really wasted."

"At this point, I can only tell you what happened to me. At first, I felt no sensation in my body. All

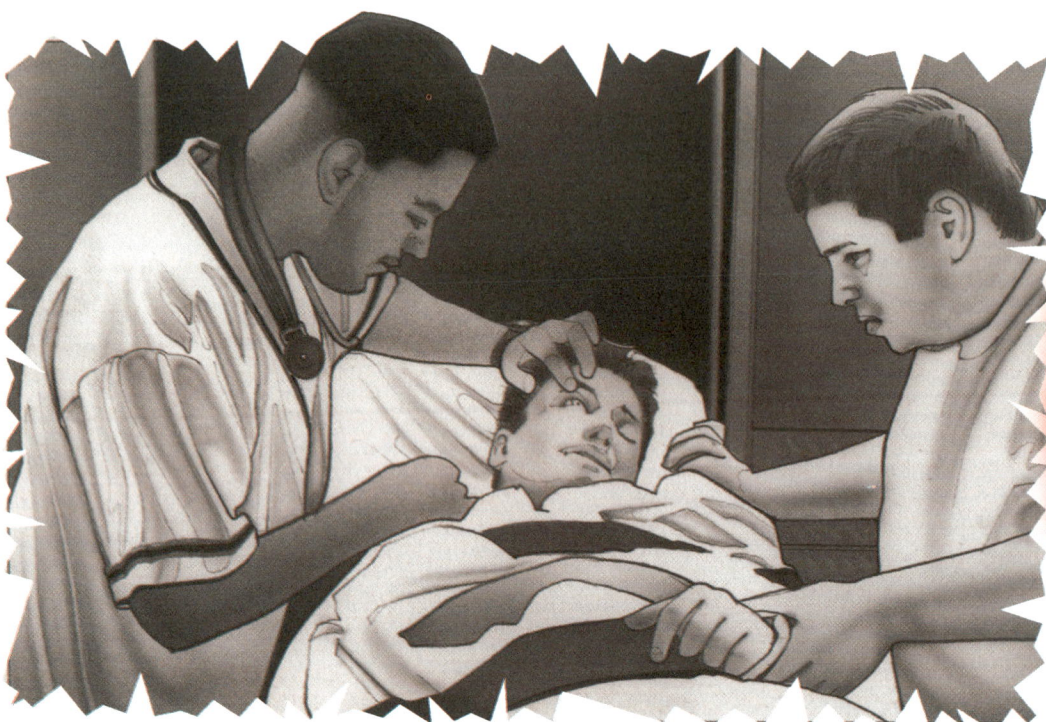

"THIS KID IS REALLY OUT OF IT."

of a sudden, everyone seemed far away. Then I felt like my brain was dying and I couldn't do anything to stop it. I started to sweat a lot; I could hear my heart beating."

"It felt like my heart was ready to jump out of my chest. I can't be certain of anything that happened afterward. I mean, everything is blank. I just can't remember."

Sharon cut in, "Well, according to the

108 HALLUCINOGENS Street Smarts

newspaper and what Mom and Dad told me, Angela's parents came home unexpectedly. When they pulled into the driveway, they heard music blasting. Some of their dishes and paintings were on the lawn. They immediately knew that there was trouble. They said that walking into their home was like walking into a scene from a horror movie. Furniture was broken and overturned, several kids were just sitting, staring into space... completely dusted. And you, you were hitting their daughter in the face and no one could pull you away."

The tears were running down Charles' face. "My own girlfriend. Why would I do such a thing?" he sobbed. "I don't want to believe that it's true, but it must be."

"It is true." Sharon added firmly, "The Kingsley's wouldn't lie. Angela's face is still swollen like a balloon and she won't talk to anyone. Your friends tell me that you just went mad."

Time For Change

"Do you remember the police and the wild ride to the hospital? "You and Angela were taken to the emergency room. The paramedics had to strap you down to control you. Luckily, some of your buddies didn't take any of your big PCP surprise, they were able to tell the doctors about the angel dust and pot that you had smoked."

"What's going to happen now?" Charles asked between sobs.

Mrs. D. got up and walked over to Charles. She had been sitting quietly in the hospital room while Sharon broke the news to Charles. She placed a hand on his shoulder and quietly said, "Sharon is right, Charles. You are lucky to be alive, so are Angela and the rest of your friends. They may never forgive you. Whether they do or not, you've got to change."

"WE HAVE THE POWER TO CHANGE OUR LIFE BY CHANGING OUR ATTITUDE OF MIND."

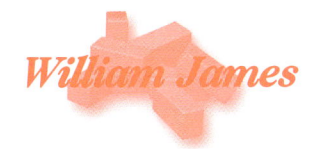

William James

TELL IT

Tripping Out

Hallucinogens are illegal mind-altering drugs. They greatly change the way the mind works. They alter the sense of sight, hearing, smell, time, and space as well as mood. They are also referred to as psychedelics.

Commonly used hallucinogens include LSD, PCP, and mescaline. They belong to a family of drugs referred to as hallucinogenics. Most hallucinogenics are made in chemical laboratories. They cause mental isolation, hallucination, and mental distortion.

LSD

Lysergic Acid Diethylamide, called LSD, Acid, Goofy, and Blot, was created in a laboratory. At first, LSD was used to study the brain and mental illness. It was found to be so dangerous that it was named an illegal substance.

Less than one drop of this powerful chemical causes severe mental changes. Since it is colorless, odorless, and tasteless, it can be added to candy or baked goods without being detected. LSD may come in pill or tablet form, in a liquid, or on small squares of blotter paper that dissolve in the mouth.

PCP

Phenylcyclidine, known as PCP, angel dust, hog, or crystal, was also developed in a laboratory. It was first used as an anesthetic during surgery and later as a tranquilizer for animals. Doctors found it so unpredictable and dangerous that it was named an illegal substance for humans.

PCP is a white powder now made in "street laboratories." The strength and ingredients vary: it may be eaten with peanut butter or added to fruit juice, or it may be swallowed, smoked, injected, sniffed, or dusted onto marijuana cigarettes. PCP is well known for causing weird or crazy behavior. Paranoia, hallucinations, and violent behavior may result from use. People have been known to jump off buildings and commit murder while under its influence.

Mescaline

Mescaline comes from the peyote cactus plant grown in Mexico and Southwestern USA. Even though it is not man-made, it causes effects similar to other hallucinogens. It is usually smoked or swallowed in tablet or capsule form.

Designer Drugs

New hallucinogenic drugs, called designer drugs, appear all the time. Designer drugs are "look-a-likes." They look like familiar hallucinogens and cause similar reactions. People who design drugs are anxious to continue making profit from drugs and to find a way to avoid arrest. These new drugs are almost the same structurally as existing illegal hallucinogens. Because they are new, they have not yet been classified as illegal. They include drugs called

STREET SMART STRATEGIES

KNOWLEDGE POWER: Learn about the dangers of hallucinogen use.

CORE VALUES: It's never too late to make positive change. Start now!

PROACTION: Take a stand—practice hallucinogen refusal skills.

BUZZ WORDS

1. Designer drug — new drugs that resemble illegal hallucinogens
2. Distortion — twisted, deformed
3. Flashback — drug experience occurring days or weeks after use of drug
4. Hallucination — seeing or hearing things that do not exist
5. Hallucinogen — substance that causes hallucination
6. LSD — (*Lysergic Acid Diethylamide*) hallucinogenic drug
7. Mescaline — hallucinogen from the peyote cactus plant
8. Paranoia — false feelings of persecution or grandeur
9. PCP — phenylcyclidine; hallucinogenic drug
10. Psychedelic — drug that causes extreme mental changes
11. Street laboratory — place where drugs are made illegally
12. Trip — slang term for a drug experience, usually involving hallucinations

Show It

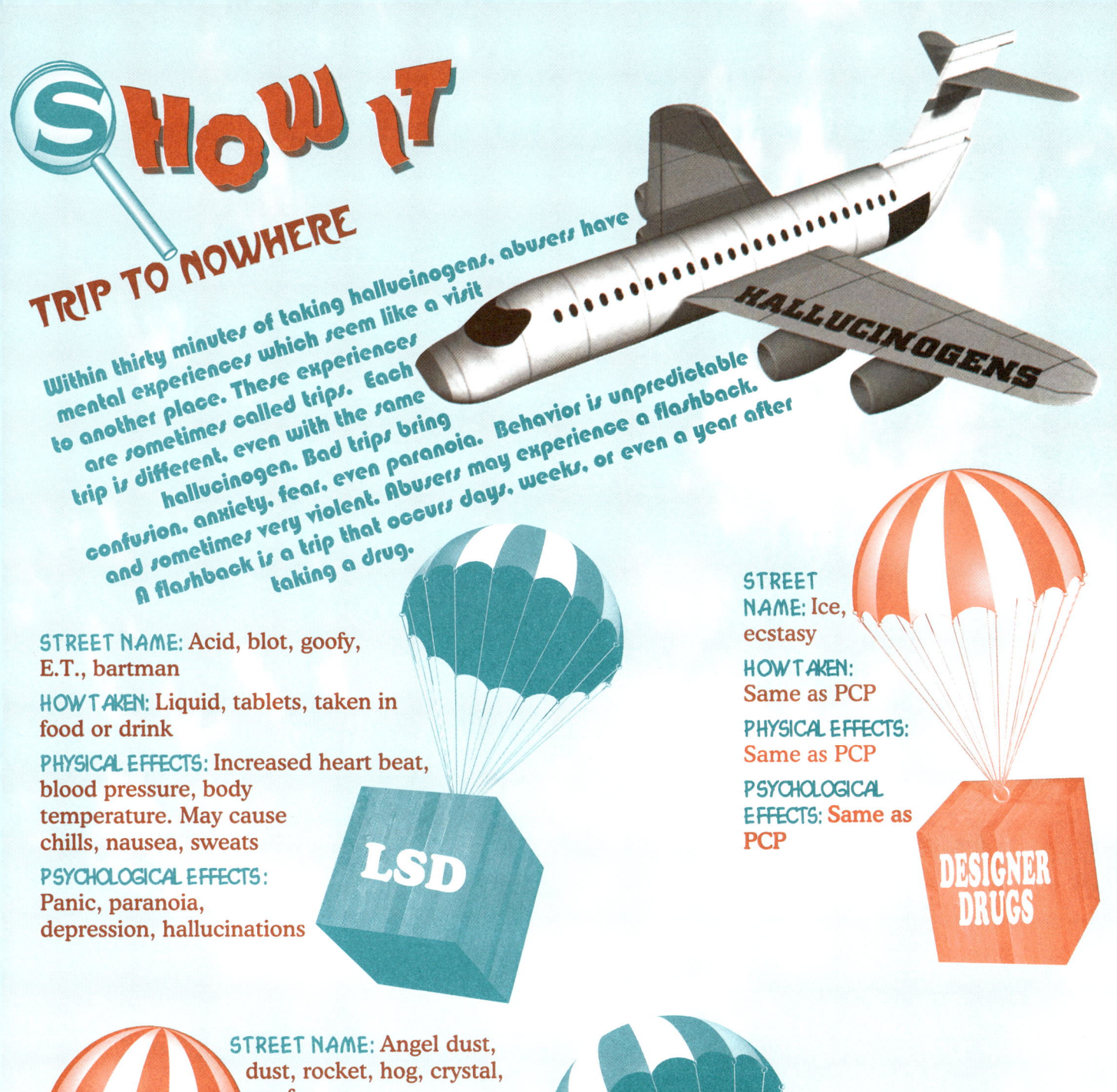

Trip to Nowhere

Within thirty minutes of taking hallucinogens, abusers have mental experiences which seem like a visit to another place. These experiences are sometimes called trips. Each trip is different, even with the same hallucinogen. Bad trips bring confusion, anxiety, fear, even paranoia. Behavior is unpredictable and sometimes very violent. Abusers may experience a flashback. A flashback is a trip that occurs days, weeks, or even a year after taking a drug.

LSD
STREET NAME: Acid, blot, goofy, E.T., bartman
HOW TAKEN: Liquid, tablets, taken in food or drink
PHYSICAL EFFECTS: Increased heart beat, blood pressure, body temperature. May cause chills, nausea, sweats
PSYCHOLOGICAL EFFECTS: Panic, paranoia, depression, hallucinations

Designer Drugs
STREET NAME: Ice, ecstasy
HOW TAKEN: Same as PCP
PHYSICAL EFFECTS: Same as PCP
PSYCHOLOGICAL EFFECTS: Same as PCP

PCP
STREET NAME: Angel dust, dust, rocket, hog, crystal, surfer
HOW TAKEN: Powder, tablets, capsules, liquid and smoked, swallowed, sniffed, or dusted onto marijuana cigarettes
PHYSICAL EFFECTS: Numbness, speeds up heart rate and blood pressure, causes sweating, slurred speech, dizziness, convulsions
PSYCHOLOGICAL EFFECTS: Violent behavior; causes anxiety, confusion, panic attacks, withdawn feelings, memory loss, poor concentration and judgement

Mescaline
STREET NAME: Mesc, peyote
HOW TAKEN: Tablet, capsule
PHYSICAL EFFECTS: Similar to LSD
PSYCHOLOGICAL EFFECTS: Similar to LSD

THE PEOPLES PUBLISHING GROUP, 1-800-822-1080. COPYING PROHIBITED BY LAW.

HOOK, LINE, AND SINKER

HOOK: The drugs that get people hooked. **LINE:** The lie that gets them to take the drugs. **SINKER:** The bad results of taking drugs.

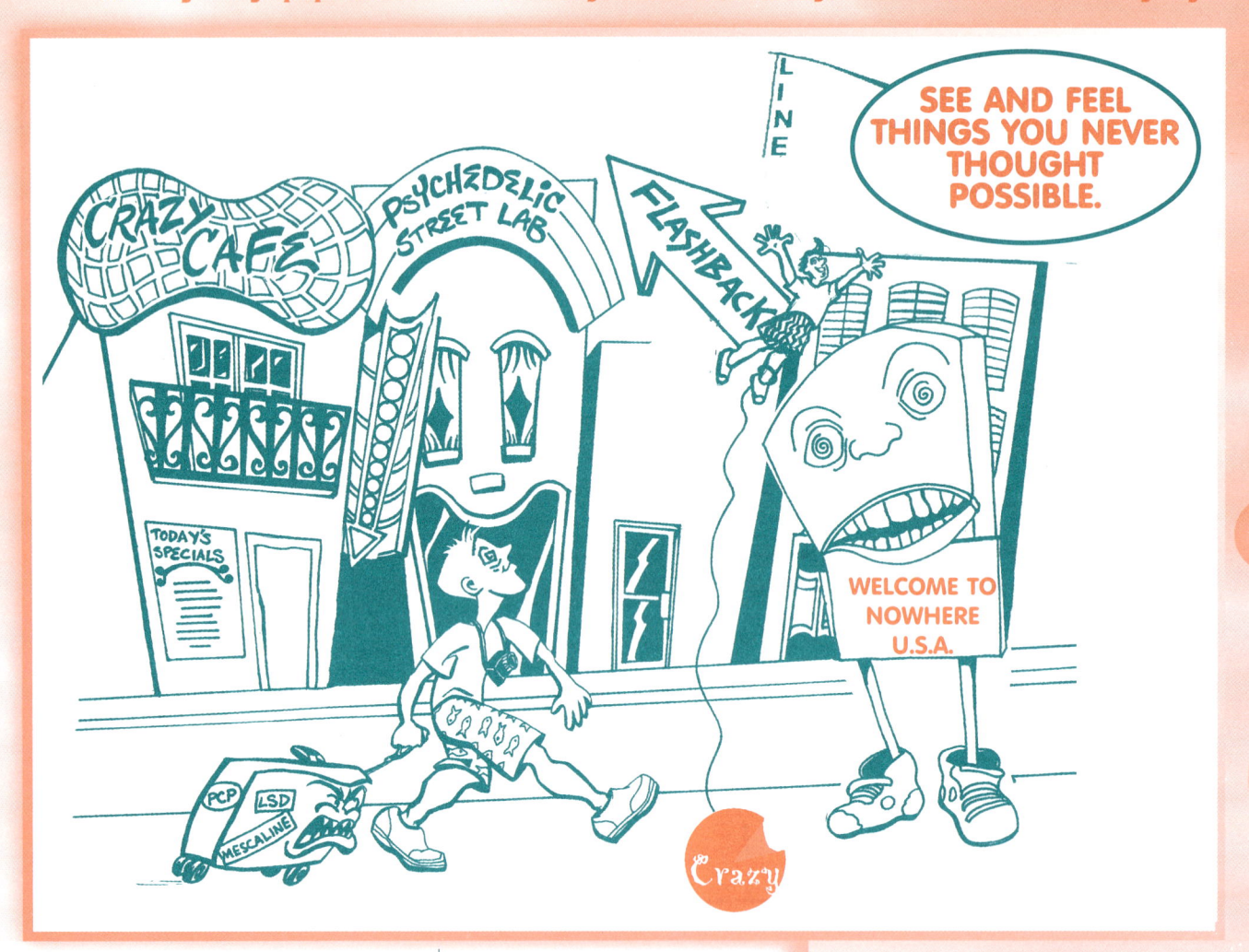

SEE AND FEEL THINGS YOU NEVER THOUGHT POSSIBLE.

THINK ABOUT IT...

Use the cartoon above to answer the following questions:

HOOK: List two hallucingens that can cause a bad trip.

LINE: How are teens enticed to abuse hallucinogens?

SINKER: What is one way an abuser might act from a flashback?

Be Street Smart

Hallucinogens are difficult to detect.

Watch carefully what you drink, eat, or smoke.

For Advice And Information Call:

National Council on Alcoholism and Drug Dependence (NCADD)

1-800-NCA-Call

or

http://www.ncadd.org

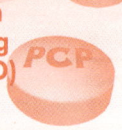

112   HALLUCINOGENS   Street Smarts

CHECKUP

MATCHING

Column A	Column B
1. ___ angel dust	a. mescaline
2. ___ acid	b. to be alone
3. ___ mesc	c. LSD
4. ___ isolated	d. frightening drug experience
5. ___ bad trip	e. PCP

FILL IN THE BLANKS

PCP   violent   psychedelics   illegal   medical   LSD   destructive   mescaline

Hallucinogens may also be called _____ because they change the way the mind works. They are _____ drugs that have no _____ use. Three hallucinogens are: _____, _____, and _____. All three can cause _____ or _____ behavior.

MULTIPLE CHOICE

1. Another name for LSD is:
a. angel dust
b. acid
c. crystal

2. Which of the following hallucinogens comes from the peyote cactus plant?
a. mescaline
b. LSD
c. PCP

3. A drug "trip" without having taken a drug is called:
a. journey
b. flashback
c. isolation

4. Angel dust, crystal, hog are street names for:
a. mescaline
b. LSD
c. PCP

5. Hallucinogens are:
a. used in surgery
b. illegal
c. legal

TAKE A STAND

Dear Mrs. D.

IMPROVE YOUR REFUSAL SKILLS

Dear Mrs. D.:

My older brother, John, does a lot of reading. He says that PCP was first developed to use with humans. He says that scientists wouldn't make something that is dangerous.

He has smoked some pot before, but now he says he wants a new kick. He wants to try some PCP to see what it is like.

Since I'm only his younger brother, he doesn't think I know anything. I do know that PCP is very dangerous. I have read several books about the violent things PCP abusers have done.

How can I get him to listen to me?

Signed,
Not too young to know better.

Write how you would answer if you were Mrs. D.

Mrs. D. Answers:

_____
_____
_____
_____
_____
_____
_____
_____
_____

Show that you recognize the danger by completing the exercise below.

Andre has no friends. He spends a lot of time by himself and feels very lonely. Each day, on his way home from school, he cuts though the park where "the heads" party on drugs. They usually ignore Andre. Andre tries to ignore them.

Yesterday one of the heads walked up to Andre, put a "duster" in Andre's mouth and said, "Come on, Andre, some 'dust' will lighten you up."

1. <u>Underline</u> a sentence that shows how Andre's feelings puts him at risk.

2. (Circle) a sentence that shows how Andre's location put him risk.

3. Write one way that Andre could meet drug-free friends.
_____
_____
_____
_____

Write the coolest way to say, "No!"

1. **The Offer** "Wanda, I have some acid. Let's take a short 'trip' together."

   You say _____
   _____

2. **The Dare** "James isn't afraid to try some dust. You're not afraid to join him, are you?"

   You say _____
   _____

   BACK OFF

3. **The Threat** "You had better take a little mesc or I'll make up a story to tell your mother about what we did."

   You say _____
   _____

4. **The Feel Good Approach** "You complain that you're bored — a little acid will make life interesting. You'll feel like you're flying."

   You say _____
   _____

114 HALLUCINOGENS Street Smarts

YOUR TURN

SPEAK OUT

LIGHTS, CAMERA, ACTION!

1. The media reports stories of violent neighborhood crimes daily: most are drug-related. How can we help to make our communities safer places to live?

_____
_____

2. Since many hallucinogenic drugs are colorless, odorless, and tasteless, how can you stay safe and certain that no one is giving you a drug?

_____
_____
_____

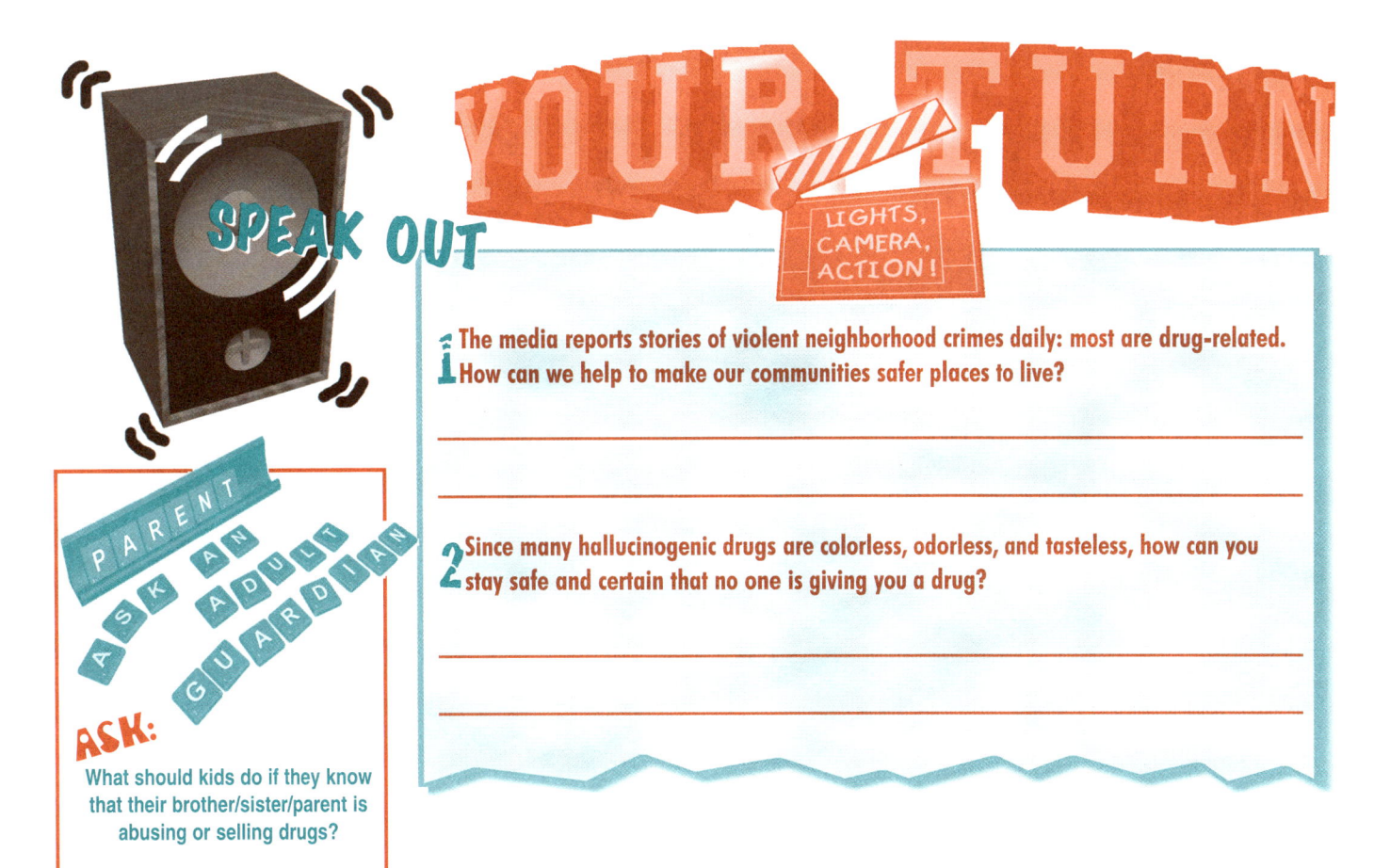

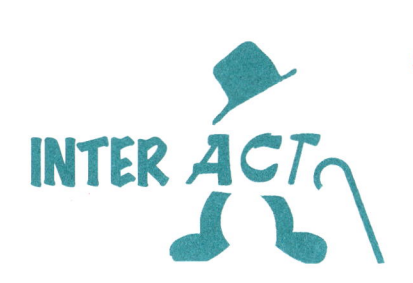

ASK A PARENT AN ADULT GUARDIAN

ASK: What should kids do if they know that their brother/sister/parent is abusing or selling drugs?

INTERACT

Setting: You are a reporter for your school newspaper.

Situation: You have heard that local all night "dance clubs" look the other way at drug use. Recently, there has been talk of kids mixing hallucinogens with soda. Some kids are also "dropping" acid into other kids' drinks. You feel that the student body should be alerted to both the danger from the club's "look the other way" attitude as well as the drugs.

Solution: How should the newspaper alert students? Tell what you will report in your article.

Teen Talk

1. Many teen drug dealers can afford the latest designer fashions. Since high school students are so conscious of "looking good," how can the dealers be made to look less desirable so that other students don't try to be like them?

_____
_____
_____
_____

2. What can schools do to promote a "drug-free" environment for their students?

_____
_____
_____
_____

THE PEOPLES PUBLISHING GROUP, 1-800-822-1080. COPYING PROHIBITED BY LAW.

GLOSSARY

A

AA Alcoholics Anonymous - help group for alcoholics
Abstain (AHB-stain) - not do something
Adrenaline (Ah-dren-UH-lynn) - hormone produced by adrenal glands that gives extra energy
Aerosols (AIR-uh-solls) - a gaseous suspension of fine solid or liquid particles
Aggressive (Uh-GRES-ive) - hostile; striking out at someone or something
Agitation (ah-juh-TAY-shun) - upset
AIDS Acquired Immune Deficiency Syndrome
Alanon (AL-uh-non) - group for family members affected by alcoholics
Alateen (AL-uh-teen) - help group for teens with alcoholic parents
Alcoholic (AL-ka-hall-ik) - a drink that contains ethyl alcohol, an addicting drug; someone who is addicted to alcohol
Alcohol poisoning (AL-ka-hall poy-sun-ing) - shuts off oxygen to the brain
Allergies (AL-ler-gees) - body's negative reaction to a substance
Amphetamines (am-FEH-tuh-mins) - stimulate or speed up body functions
Anabolic steroid (ann-uh-BOHL-ik ster-oyd) - chemical taken internally to promote weight gain and muscle growth
Analgesic (ann-uhl-GEE-zic) - pain killer; substance that numbs
Anxiety (ang-XI-it-ee) - a feeling of tension, stress, or worry
Artificial (ar-tah-FISH-ul) - not natural; man-made
Aversion therapy (uh-VER-shun THER-uh-pee) - makes smoking unpleasant so smokers avoid smoking

B

BAL or blood alcohol level - measure of the amount of alcohol in a person's blood
Barbiturates (bar-bi-chur-it) - drugs that depress or slow down body functions
Binge (binj) - to over-indulge in something
Blanks (blanx) - slang for "false" steroids
Bong (bong) - pipe used to produce a stronger effect from marijuana
Breathing (bree-thing) - taking in oxygen, pushing out carbon dioxides
Burn out (BURN out) - term used to describe a person who uses a lot of marijuana and who lacks interest in life

C

Cannabis sativa plant (CAN-uh-bus sah-TEE-va plant) - marijuana plant
Carbon monoxide CAR-bin mon-OX-eyed) - a colorless, odorless, poison gas that replaces oxygen in the lungs
Cartel (CAR-tell) - an association of drug producers and sellers that set prices and control the drug market
Carcinogenic (car-SIN-o-jen-ik) - cancer-causing
Chewing tobacco (CHU-ing tah-BACK-oh) - tobacco placed between the gums an the teeth and chewed
Chug (chug) - drink heavily
Cocaine (KO-kane) - illegal drug made from coca leaves; powder called "coke" or "snow"
Cold turkey (kold TUR-kee) - method of quitting smoking by just stopping
Coordinate (co-OR-din-eight) - work together
Convulsions (con-VUL-shun) - uncontrollable body movements
Cut (kut) - to dilute or add "fillers" to stretch a drug
Crack (krak) - a "rock" form of cocaine that can be smoked
Crack babies (krak BAY-bees) - children born to mothers who smoked crack
Crack house (krak hous) - place where users go to buy and smoke crack
Crash (krash) - the low feeling or depression present when the drug wears off

D

Dealer (DEEL-er) - person who sells drugs
Deformities (Dee-FORM-it-ees) - parts of the body not formed properly
Deny (DIH-ni) - to pretend that a problem does not exist
Dependence (DIH-pen-dens) - relying or counting on someone or something
Dependent (DIH-pen-dehnt) - unable to do without; to rely on something
Depressant (DIH-pres-sent) - slows down body functions
Depression (dih-PRES-shun) - continued feeling of intense sadness
Designer drug (dih-SIHN-er druhg) - new drugs that resemble illegal hallucinogens
Distilled (DIHS-tild) - process of heating that makes alcohol stronger, such as whiskey or vodka
Distortion (DIHS-tore-shun) - twisted, deformed
Downers (DOUN-er) - depressants; drugs that slow down body functions
Drug (druhg) - alters the way cells and tissues in the body work
Drug abuse (druhg AH-buys) - misuse of any drug
Drug lord (druhg lord) - most powerful person who controls the drug business
Drug reactions (druhg ree-AX-shuns) - the body's response to a drug
Drunk (drungk) - under the influence of alcohol
Dual or cross-addiction (do-al kros-uh-DIKT-shun) - to be addicted to more than one drug

E

Ecstasy (X-tih-cee) - street name for illegal amphetamine type drug
Enabling behaviors (en-A-bell-ing BEE-hav-yurs) - excuses made up by friends and families for the inappropriate actions of an alcoholic
Endorphin (ehn-DOOR-fin) - natural chemical produced by the body; allows person to feel natural highs and lows
Euphoria (u-FOR-e-uh) - a feeling of great happiness or well-being
Exhale (X-hail) - breathe out
Expired (X-pired) - finished; should no longer be used
Expiration date (x-per-A-shun date) - when the medicine should no longer be used

F

Fermented (FER-men-tid) - process of using yeast with grains and fruits to make alcoholic beverages, such as beer or wine
Flashback (FLASH-bak) - interruption of the present by a memory of the past
Freebase (FREE-base) - smokable form of cocaine
Fumes (fyoomz) - gases or vapors given off by chemicals

G

Gateway drug (GATE-way druhg) - a drug that leads addicts to using other drugs
Glamorize (GLAM-or-eyes) - to make something seem special

H

Hallucinogen (huh-LOU-zen-a-jen) - substance that causes hallucination
Hallucinations (huh-loo-zen-A-shuns) - thoughts and fantasies that appear to be real
Hangover (HANG-o-ver) - sick feeling; result of drinking too much
Hash (hash) - string form of marijuana made from resin of plant
Hepatitis (hep-uh-TI-tis) - a liver disease spread through the exchange of blood
Heroin (HER-oh-in) - a highly addictive drug made from the seeds of a poppy plant
Hit (hit) - amount of drug taken
Hooked (hookt) - dependent; addicted to a drug
Hormone (HOR-moan) - chemical made by the glands of the body
Hyperactive (hi-per-AK-tive) - very active
Hypochondriac (hi-per-CON-dree-ak) - someone who imagines illness and may cause themselves to become sick
Hypnosis (hip-NO-sis) - method of quitting smoking using the power of suggestion

I

Immune system (E-myoon SIS-tem) - the body's defense system that helps fight invading germs
Impotence (im-PUH-tence) - inability to have sex
Inappropriate (in-uh-PRO-pree-it) - not proper
Infertile (in-FUR-tl) - unable to have children

Inhale (IN-hail) - breathe into the lungs
Inhalant (in-HAIL-int) - substances with fumes inhaled for a special effect
Insomnia (in-SOM-nee-a) - inability to sleep
Interfere (IN-ter-fear) - to prevent or get in the way of
Intoxicating (in-TOKS-sih-kat-ing) - causing a person to get drunk
Invade (IN-vade) - to attack
IV drug (intravenous drug) - drug that us taken through a vein

J

Joint (joint) - dried leaves, buds, or flowers of the marijuana plant that is rolled and smoked like a cigarette
Joy rider (joi ride) - person who abuses steroids

L

Liquor (LICK-er) - stronger alcohol than wine or beer because much of the water is taken out of the alcohol
LSD (Lysergic Acid Diethylamide) (el-es-dee) - hallucinogenic drug

M

Mainline (MAIN-line) - to inject heroin into a vein with a needle
Medical history (med-i-KEL HEH-stor-ee) - a record of medical illnesses and conditions that you have or once had
Medicine (MED-e-sin) - a drug prescribed by a doctor or an over-the-counter drug taken for health reasons
Mescaline (MESK-uh-lin) - hallucinogen from the peyote cactus plant
Methadone (METH-uh-dohn) - legal, man-made addictive drug sometimes used in the treatment of heroin addicts
Methamphetamines (meth-uh-FET-uh-mins) - an illegal amphetamine-type drug
Motivation (moh-tuh-VA-shun) - determination or will to do something

N

Nausea (naw-ZEE-uh) - feeling sick to your stomach
Nicotine (nic-UH-teen) - a chemical causing the desire for tobacco
Nicotine fit (nic-UH-teen fit) - an addicted person's body demands nicotine; person feels like they must have tobacco

O

Overdose (O-ver-dos) - to take too much of
Over-the-counter (OTC) - legal drugs sold without prescription in a pharmacy

P

Paranoia (par-uh-NOY-ah) - false feelings of persecution or grandeur
Passive smoking (PASS-ive SMOK-ng) - non-smoker who breathes in second-hand smoke
PCP (Phenylcyclidine) - hallucinogenic drug
Pharmacist (FARM-uh-cist) - trained professional who fills prescriptions
Physician's Desk Reference (PDR) - reference book that describes medical products and possible reactions
Potency (POH-ten-cee) - strength of a drug
Prescribed (PRE-skribed) - medicine ordered by a doctor with a doctor's note
Prescription (Pre-SKRIP-shun) - note from a medical doctor for a particular medicine
Problem drinker (PROB-lem DRINK-er) - someone who is dependent on alcohol
Prostitution (Pros-teh-TU-shun) - sale of body in exchange for something
Psychedelic (siik-uh-DELL-ik) - drug that causes extreme mental changes

R

Rate of Absorption - time it takes for alcohol to get into your blood
Resin (RES-in) - sticky substance from leaves or flowers of a marijuana plant
Ripped (Rehpt) - increased muscle definition of body builder
Roach clip (rooch klip) - holder for a marijuana cigarette in order to smoke it to a small butt
Rock (rok) - slang for "crack"
Roid rages (royd rage) - uncontrolled burst of anger due to the abuse of steroids
Runs (runs) - repeated or continual drug use to avoid the "crash
Rush (rush) - an intense feeling of pleasure

S

SADD - Students Against Destructive Decisions
Seedpod (SEED-pod) - part of plant that holds and protects the seeds
Shooting gallery (SHU-ting GALL-er-ee) - place where abusers go to inject themselves with heroin
Side-stream smoke (SIID-stream smoke) - secondhand smoke; smoke-filled air around a smoker
Skinpop (skin-POP) - to inject heroin under the surface of the skin
Smokeless tobacco (smok-less tih-back-oh)- tobacco sniffed, chewed or held in mouth, but not smoked
Snuff (snuff) - finely ground tobacco sniffed through nostrils or held against gums
Snort (snort) - to inhale through the nose
Snorting (SNORT-ing) - inhaling heroin through the nose
Sober (SO-ber) - not drunk
Social drinker (SO-shul DRINK-er) - someone who drinks with others on special occasions
Solitude (SOL-ih-tude) - alone; away from others
STD - Sexually Transmitted Disease
Sterile (STER-uhl) - unable to produce children
Sterility (ster-ILL-it-ee) - inability to have children
Stimulant (STIM-u-lent) - a drug that speeds up body activities such as heartbeat
Stoned (stoned) - high; intoxicated on marijuana
Street drug (STREET-druhg) - illegal drug; non-medical drug sold on the street
Street laboratory (street lab-or-ah-TOR-ee) - place where drugs are made illegally
Stroke (STROKUH)- condition in which brain and nerve tissue die due to poor blood supply. This may cause loss of speech or paralysis.
Stunted (STUN-ted)- prevented from growing or developing properly
Suffocation (suf-fih-KA-shun)- to die from a lack of oxygen
Suspicious (suh-PISH-us)- feeling mistrust
Symptoms (SIMP-tums) - signs that your body gives when your system is out of balance
Synthetic (sin-THE-tik) - not natural; man-made

T

Testosterone (tes-TOS-ter-own) - male hormone
THC (tetrahydrocannabinol) - mind-altering chemical in marijuana
Tolerance (TOL-ehr-ence) - ability to withstand more of a drug without feeling the effects
Toxic (TOX-ik) - poison
Tranquilizer (tran-quill-I-zer) - a calming drug
Trip (TRIP) - slang term used for a drug experience, usually involving hallucinations

U

Uppers (UH-pers) - slang for amphetamine

V

Ventilated (ven-till-A-ted) - getting fresh air
Vial (VI-uhl) - plastic container from which crack is sold

W

Weed (WEED) - slang expression for marijuana
Withdrawal (with-DRAW-uhl) - powerful symptoms that occur when abuser stops using drug

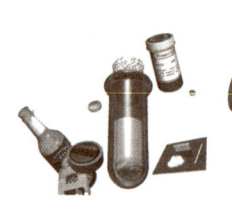

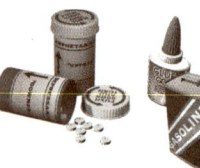

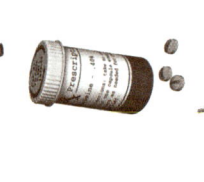

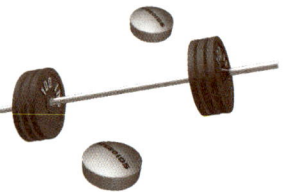

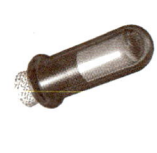

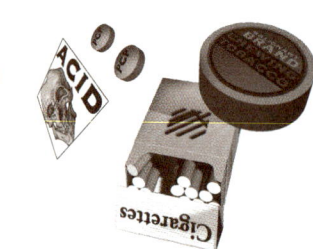

INDEX

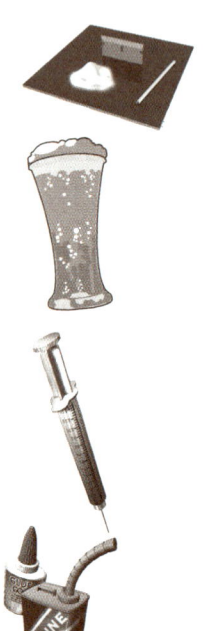

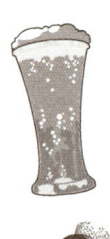

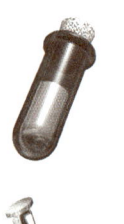

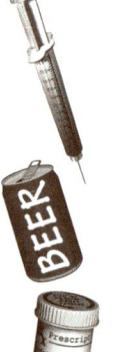

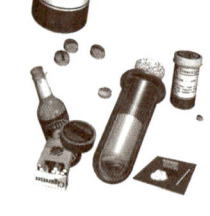

AIDS, 22, 23, 49, 58, 65, 74
AA, 22
Alanon, 22, 26
Alateen, 22, 26
Alcohol, 11-19, 20-30
Amphetamines/Depressants, 81-98
   adrenaline, 83
   barbiturates, 83
   behaviours, 83
   dual addiction, 84
   effects of, 85
   methamphetamines, 83
   physical response, 83
   tranquilizers, 83
Blood Alochol Level, 14
   cycle of addiction, 14
   effects of, 13
   enabling behaviours, 25
   fermenting, 13
   levels of dependence, 22
   physical effects, 24
   psychological effects, 24
   rate of absorption, 15
   tolerance, 15
Cocaine, 55-62
   abusers, 58
   crash, 58
   craving, 58
   dealers, 57
   effects of, 57
   freebase, 57
   high, 58
   history of, 57
Crack, 63-71
   addiction, 65, 67
   babies, 67
   binges, 65
   crash, 65
   dependence, 65
   fatality, 67
   physical effects, 66
   production, 65
   psychological effects, 66
Drugs, 1-10
   abuse, 5
   abusers, 5
   behaviours of abuse, 4
   early use, 4
   finding help, 4
   overdose, 4
   present use, 4
   street drugs, 4
   testing, 67
   uses and abuses, 4
Hallucinogens, 108-115
   designer drugs, 110
   LSD, PCP, 110
   Mescaline, 110
   methods of use, 111
   physical effects, 111
   psychological effects, 111
Heroin, 72-80
   addiction, 76
   drug cartel/lord, 74
   endorphins, 75
   hepatitis, 74
   highs, 75
   IV drug, 74
   mainlining/skinpopping/snorting, 74
   physical effects, 76
   psychological effects, 76
   shooting gallery, 74
   snorting, 74
   withdrawal, 75
Inhalants, 90-98
   aerosols, 92
   dangers of, 93
   effects, 92, 94
   examples of, 94
   methods of use, 94
   physical/psychological effects, 94
   respiration, 92
   symtoms, 94
Marijuana, 39-46
   effects of, 42
   forms of, 41
   hash, 41
   methods of use, 41
   physical effects, 42
NCAPP, 7
Over-the-counter/Prescription drugs, 99-107
   body responses, 103
   bulimia, 100
   healthy habits, 103
   immune, 101
   medicine labels, 102
   over-the-counter drugs, 101
   working with doctors, 102
SADD, 13
   Contract for life, iii, iv
STD, 22, 23, 74
Steroids, 47-54
   anabolic, 49
   blanks, 50
   testosterone, 49
Tobacco, 30-38
   addiction, 32
   carbon monoxide, 32
   effects of quitting, 33
   fatalities, 32
   five ways to quit, 34
   nicotine, 32
   passive smoking, 32
   secondhand smoke, 32
   smokeless tobacco, 32

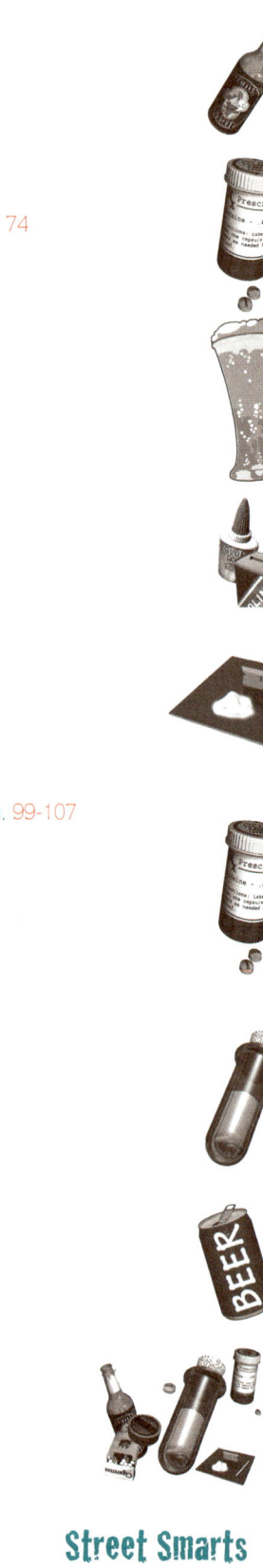

Personal Growth Worksheet

Join the STREET SMARTS team. Send us your best *Situation, Strategy* and *Support* ideas for developing drug refusal skills. Your ideas, experiences and "Street Smarts" strategies can help others by encouraging drug-free living.

Send To:
Dr. June Stride & Richard Wolf
The Peoples Publishing Group, Inc.
230 W. Passaic Street
Maywood, New Jersey 07607

PRACTICE YOUR REFUSAL SKILLS

SITUATION
(Describe risk for substance abuse.)
_____
_____
_____

STRATEGY
(List positive steps for drug-proofing the situaiton. Write your response.)
_____
_____
_____

SUPPORT
(List family, friends, organizations that can assist you in remaining drug-free.)
_____
_____
_____

THE PEOPLES PUBLISHING GROUP, 1-800-822-1080. COPYING PROHIBITED BY LAW.

Personal Growth Worksheet

Join the **STREET SMARTS** team. Send us your best *Situation, Strategy* and *Support* ideas for developing drug refusal skills. Your ideas, experiences and "Street Smarts" strategies can help others by encouraging drug-free living.

Send To:
Dr. June Stride & Richard Wolf
The Peoples Publishing Group, Inc.
230 W. Passaic Street
Maywood, New Jersey 07607

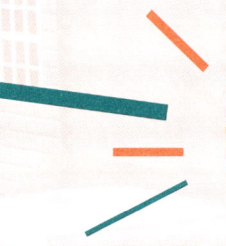

PRACTICE YOUR REFUSAL SKILLS

SITUATION
(Describe risk for substance abuse.)

_____
_____
_____

STRATEGY
(List positive steps for drug-proofing the situation. Write your response.)

_____
_____
_____

SUPPORT
(List family, friends, organizations that can assist you in remaining drug-free.)

_____
_____
_____